COMMON LABORATORY
TESTS USED BY TCM
PRACTITIONERS

of related interest

Acupuncture for New Practitioners
John Hamwee
ISBN 978 1 84819 102 0
eISBN 978 0 85701 083 4

Basic Theories of Traditional Chinese Medicine
Edited by Zhu Bing and Wang Hongcai
ISBN 978 1 84819 038 2
eISBN 978 0 85701 020 9
Part of the International Acupuncture Textbooks series

Diagnostics of Traditional Chinese Medicine
Edited by Zhu Bing and Wang Hongcai
ISBN 978 1 84819 036 8
eISBN 978 0 85701 019 3
Part of the International Acupuncture Textbooks series

Pocket Handbook of Particularly Effective Acupoints for Common Conditions Illustrated in Color
Guo Changqing Guoyan and Zhaiwei Liu Naigang
ISBN 978 1 84819 120 4
eISBN 978 0 85701 094 0

Pocket Handbook of Body Reflex Zones Illustrated in Color
Guo Changqing Guoyan and Zhaiwei Liu Naigang
ISBN 978 1 84819 119 8
eISBN 978 0 85701 095 7

COMMON LABORATORY TESTS USED BY TCM PRACTITIONERS

When to Refer Patients for Lab Tests and How to Read and Interpret the Results

Partha Banerjee, MD and Christina Captain, DOM

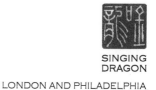

SINGING
DRAGON

LONDON AND PHILADELPHIA

First published in 2014
by Singing Dragon
an imprint of Jessica Kingsley Publishers
73 Collier Street
London N1 9BE, UK
and
400 Market Street, Suite 400
Philadelphia, PA 19106, USA

www.singingdragon.com

Library of Congress Cataloging in Publication Data
Banerjee, Partha, 1945- author.
Common laboratory tests used by TCM practitioners :
when to refer patients for lab tests and how to
read and interpret the results / Partha Banerjee and Christina Captain.
p. ; cm.
Includes bibliographical references and index.
ISBN 978-1-84819-205-8 (alk. paper) -- ISBN 978-0-85701-164-0
I. Captain, Christina, 1967- author. II. Title.
[DNLM: 1. Clinical Laboratory Techniques--Handbooks.
2. Clinical Laboratory Techniques--Problems
and Exercises. 3. Clinical Laboratory Services--Handbooks.
4. Clinical Laboratory Services--Problems and
Exercises. 5. Medicine, Chinese Traditional--Handbooks.
6. Medicine, Chinese Traditional--Problems
and Exercises. QY 39]
RT48
616.07'5--dc23
2013048143

British Library Cataloguing in Publication Data
A CIP catalogue record for this book is available from the British Library

ISBN 978 1 84819 205 8
eISBN 978 0 85701 164 0

Printed and bound in Great Britain

For my mother

CONTENTS

PREFACE

This handbook of laboratory testing is specifically prepared for students and practitioners of Traditional Chinese Medicine (TCM). As integrated medical teams all over the world are learning to work as cohesive units, it is important that TCM practitioners become competent with the basics of laboratory analysis.

We are pleased to see the growing number of TCM practitioners who are ordering, interpreting, and, in general, using more laboratory testing in the treatment of their patients. Our hope is that this handbook will help to bridge the gap between Eastern and Western schools of medicine and improve the overall care of the patient, which is the ultimate goal.

Special effort has been made to keep this text concise and to deal with subject matter that is pertinent to the practitioner of TCM. Comprehensive details of laboratory testing, especially related to inpatient care and acute care situations have been intentionally excluded. For those who are interested, additional information can easily be found in standard laboratory textbooks. This handbook will serve to introduce practitioners of TCM to common laboratory tests and help them communicate more effectively with various practitioners of conventional medicine.

You will find the format of this book to be different from most other texts. Rather than tests being tabulated and described alphabetically, the laboratory tests in this book are grouped together as they pertain to diseases or systems. For example, in the chapter on diabetes and glucose metabolism, the tests are arranged as they may be needed when treating a patient with diabetes mellitus.

At the end of each chapter there is a TCM perspective summary, the goal of which is to provide a basic scenario of when, why, and how to utilize conventional laboratory testing within a TCM practice. It does not serve to list all of the TCM symptoms or to identify a TCM pattern. The term "best practice" is utilized to identify a pathway of action that indicates the superior decision related to the management of patients by a TCM practitioner. Best practices will ultimately become a basis for the development of the standard of practice for TCM practitioners all over the world. The term "evidence base" is used to identify when we should acquire baseline documentation in order to show progress or to justify a course of treatment.

It is our intention that this handbook will be a useful tool for TCM students and practitioners and that it supports and encourages an integrated approach to doing what is best for our patients.

LIST OF ABBREVIATIONS

ACE inhibitor Angiotensin-converting-enzyme inhibitor

ACTH Adrenocorticotropic hormone

ADH Anti-diuretic hormone

ALT Alanine aminotransferase

ASHD Atherosclerotic heart diseases

AST Aspartate transaminase

AVP Arginine vasopressin (antidiuretic hormone)

BUN Blood urea nitrogen

CBC Complete blood count

CHF Congestive heart failure

COPD Chronic obstructive pulmonary disease

CT Computerized tomography

ER Emergency room

ETOH Ethanol

FH Family history

FSH Follicle stimulating hormone

G6PD Glucose-6-phosphate dehydrogenase deficiency

GAD Glutamic acid decarboxylase

GFR Glomerular filtration rate

GGT Gamma-glutamyltransferase

GI Gastrointestinal

HbA1c Glycated hemaglobin

HDP High density lipoprotein

HPI History of present illness

ICA Islet cell auto-antibodies

IM Intramuscular

IV Intravenous

LDH Lactate dehydrogenase

LDL Low density lipoprotein

LH Luteinizing hormone

MCH Mean corpuscular hemoglobin

MCHC Mean cell hemoglobin concentration

MCV Mean corpuscular volume

MRI Magnetic resonance imaging

PCP Primary care physician

PE Physical exam

PH Past history

PT Prothrombin time

PTH Parathyroid hormone

PTT Partial thromboplastin time

RBC Red blood cell

RDW Red cell distribution width

RE Reticuloendothelial

SGOT Serum glutamic oxabacetic transaminase

SGPT Serum glutamic pyruvic transaminase

SH Social history

SIADH Syndrome of inappropriate antidiuretic hormone

SOB Shortness of breath

TCM Traditional Chinese medicine

TIBC Total iron binding capacity

TSH Thyroid stimulating hormone

UTI Urinary tract infection

VLDL Very low density lipoprotein

WBC White blood cell

WNL Within normal limits

1

COMPLETE BLOOD COUNT

The Complete Blood Count (CBC) is a common test that should be ordered at first contact with most new patients, and then at periodic intervals as needed.

Information that can be deduced from a CBC includes:

- Red Blood Cells Series
  - Anemia
  - Identify the kind of anemia
  - Determine changes in red cell mass/size
- White Blood Cells Series
  - Presence of infection

- ○ White blood cell (WBC) malignancies, such as leukemia
- ○ Leukemoid reaction
- ○ Leucopenia
- Platelets
  - ○ Thrombocytopenia
  - ○ Determine etiology of easy bruising or poor coagulation
  - ○ Determine etiology of low platelet count

Normal CBC Results

Hemoglobin: 11.5–15.0 g/dL

Hematocrit: 34.0–44.0%

Mean corpuscular volume (MCV): 80–98 fL ($80–98$ μm^3)

Platelets: 140–415 × 10E3/uL (140–415 10^6 × mm^3)

Leucocyte: 3.4–10.8 × 10E3/uL (3.4–10.8 10^6 × mm^3)

BASIC SCIENCE
Red Blood Cell

Normal

Male: 4–6 × 10E6/uL (4–6 10^6 × mm^3)

Female: 3.8–5.1 × 10E6/uL (3.8–5.1 10^6 × mm^3)

Red blood cells (RBCs) are made in the bone marrow. The precursor cell is called a proerythroblast, which is a large nucleated cell. With maturation the cell gets smaller, assumes a biconcave shape, and the nucleus is gradually fragmented and removed. The main function of the RBC is to carry oxygen and carbon dioxide. Normally, RBCs show no evidence of a nucleus by the time the cell is released in circulation. Cells containing the remnants of a nucleus are called reticulocytes. In a healthy individual, about 1–1.5% of the RBCs in circulation are reticulocytes. Whenever RBC production is elevated, the number of reticulocytes is increased. Increased reticulocyte counts are often seen in hemolytic anemia or after replacement with vitamin B12 or iron in a person who was vitamin B12- or iron-deficient. Reticulocyte count is decreased with bone marrow malfunction due to the decrease in total number of cells being produced.

BLOOD TESTS FOR ANEMIA

The normal function of a RBC is to transport oxygen and carbon dioxide. When the number or quality of the RBCs is reduced, the resulting diagnosis is anemia. This is a very common and important diagnosis in medical practice. The following information describes a simple approach in the diagnosis of anemia. Following this algorithm is definitely not all-inclusive, but the algorithm is practical and will be very helpful for the TCM practitioner. Initially, observe the two most important parameters, which are hemoglobin and MCV.

Hemoglobin

As described above, the normal range for hemoglobin is given as 11.5–15 g/dL. However, for practical purposes, especially when dealing with the diagnosis of anemia, the following numbers may be more helpful:

Normal

Male: 14 g/dL

Female: 11.5 g/dL

Mean Corpuscular Volume

Normal: 80–100 fL (80–100 μm³)

The MCV is the volume of a single RBC and is a very useful index in differentiating between the various types of anemias. The volume of a single RBC (average) is measured and categorized as:

- Small or microcytic (< 80 fL/<80 μm³)
- Big or macrocytic or megaloblastic (>100 fL/ >100 μm³)
- Normal or normocytic (80–100 fL/80–100 μm³)

Looking at a CBC report (see example), there are about 20 different parameters that tend to confuse students. As stated previously, you should only focus on two of these— hemoglobin and MCV.

After reviewing the CBC, some additional tests may need to be ordered separately. These are essential to determine the specific type of anemia and will be described in detail later in this chapter. The additional tests to be ordered are:

- Serum vitamin B12 level
- Serum folic acid level
- Iron level
- TIBC
- Ferritin level
- Reticulocyte count

Steps for Reviewing a CBC for Anemia

1. Check the hemoglobin value. If the hemoglobin is <14 g/dL for men or <11.5 g/dL for women, the diagnosis is anemia.

2. If step one is positive for anemia, then check the MCV value.

   ○ A value <80 fL (<80 μm³) indicates microcytic anemia.

   ○ A value >100 fL (>100 μm³) indicates macrocytic anemia (i.e., megaloblastic anemia).

   ○ A value 80–100 fL (80–100 μm³) indicates normocytic anemia.

   The etiologies of microcytic anemia are:

   ○ Iron-deficiency anemia

   ○ Anemia of chronic illness

   ○ Sideroblastic anemia (for more details see Harrison, 2011)

   The etiologies of macrocytic anemia are:

   ○ Vitamin B12 deficiency

   ○ Folic acid deficiency

   The etiologies of normocytic anemia are:

   ○ Hemolytic anemia

   ○ Bone marrow pathologies/dysfunction

   For additional information relating to the type and etiology of an anemia, second-line tests need to be ordered immediately.

3. Second-line tests for microcytic anemia are:

   ◦ Serum iron level

   ◦ Total iron binding capacity (TIBC)

   ◦ Ferritin level

   Second-line test for macrocytic anemia are:

   ◦ Vitamin B12 level

   ◦ Folic acid level

   Second-line test for normocytic anemia is:

   ◦ Reticulocyte count

   With second-line test results, the specific type of anemia can be deduced. In microcytic anemia (MCV <80 fL/<80 μm³), with second-line tests values as follows:

   ◦ If serum iron and TIBC values are low, the anemia type is indicative of chronic illness.

   ◦ If serum iron is low and TIBC is high, the anemia type is indicative of iron deficiency, further confirmed by a low or low normal ferritin value.

   Iron-deficiency anemia can generally indicate occult blood loss most commonly from menstrual or gastrointestinal (GI) tract bleeding. Due to the various locations that bleeding can occur in the body, it is best practice to order a hemoccult stool test, which will help differentiate the etiology of the bleeding (see Chapter 2).

   In macrocytic anemia (MCV>100 fL/>100 μm³), with second-line test values as follows:

   ◦ Low vitamin B12 value indicates vitamin B12 deficiency (i.e., megaloblastic anemia).

○ Low folic acid value indicates folic acid deficiency.

In normocytic anemia (MCV 80–100 fL/80–100 μm^3), with second line test values as follows:

○ Increased reticulocyte count may suggest hemolytic anemia (see below).

○ Decreased reticulocyte count may suggest bone marrow disease (see below).

The etiologies of hemolytic anemia are:

- Hemoglobinopathies (i.e., sickle cell anemia)

- Globin disorders, such as thalassemia

- Enzyme defects, such as glucose-6-phosphate dehydrogenase deficiency (G6PD) disorders

- Membrane defects, such as hereditary spherocytosis

The etiologies of bone marrow disease are:

- Aplastic anemia

- Bone marrow infiltration with malignancy

- Chemotherapy

- Exposure to toxins (e.g., benzene)

ADDITIONAL BLOOD TESTS FOR ANEMIA

Additional blood tests necessary to classify anemia after reviewing basic CBC are described below.

Vitamin B12

Normal: 200–835 pg/mL

Vitamin B12 is mainly derived from animal sources and assists in nerve conduction and the formation of RBCs.

Decreased levels are commonly seen in pernicious anemia; however, malabsorption due to disease or organ dysfunction can also contribute.

Folic Acid

Normal: 150–800 pg/mL

Normal levels of folic acid assist in the formation of RBCs. Decreased levels are often seen in barbiturate drug use and some chemotherapies.

Iron

Normal

Male: 65–175 ug/dL

Female: 50–175 ug/dL

Iron is essential for the formation of hemoglobin, which is the compound that carries oxygen and carbon dioxide. Low levels are seen in:

- Chronic blood loss, usually GI bleed or heavy menstrual blood loss
- Habitual blood donor
- Iron-deficient diet
- Parasitic infestation (e.g., hook worm)

High levels are seen in:

- Hemochromatosis

Total Iron Binding Capacity

Normal: 259–1000 ug/dL

This test is useful in determining the cause of microcytic anemia. Decreased levels are seen in:

- Anemia of chronic illness

Increased levels are seen in:

- Iron-deficiency anemia

Ferritin

Ferritin is an excellent indicator of iron stores in the body, and therefore assessing serum ferritin gives a more accurate indication of iron deficiency than serum iron. Unfortunately, ferritin is also an acute phase reactant and increases with stress and inflammation, which can make it difficult to assess accurately.

Normal

Male: 20–270 ng/mL

Female: 20–170 ng/mL

Decreased levels are seen in:

- Iron-deficiency anemia

Increased levels are seen in:

- Hemochromatosis
- Inflammation

White Blood Cell

Normal: 4.0–10.5 × 10E3/uL (4000–10,500/mm^3)

There are five different classifications of white blood cells (WBCs), which are divided into two groups:

1. Granulocytes: neutrophils, eosinophils, and basophils

2. Agranulocytes: lymphocytes and monocytes

WBCs are formed in the bone marrow, as are red blood cells, but the functions are different. Their main function is defense; they destroy infectious organisms and cancer cells either by phagocytosis or by producing antibodies.

Note: Many African American adults have a lower and cyclically changing WBC count.

Increased leukocyte count may have any of the following etiologies:

- Bacterial infection: Total WBC count is raised two- or three-fold.

- Leukemoid reaction: In some infections, the WBC count is temporarily raised to levels high enough to suggest the possibility of leukemia. The temporary character and some chemical features (leukocyte alkaline phosphatase) help differentiate these other infections from leukemia.

- Leukemia, all classifications.

- Many types of cancer.

Leucopenia (WBC <4000) may indicate:

- Viral infection

- Bone marrow pathology/dysfunction

- Hypersplenism

- Auto-immune conditions

DIFFERENTIAL COUNT

In a differential count of WBCs, each of the five classifications of WBC is counted individually and their number is expressed as a ratio to the total WBC count.

Increased neutrophils may indicate:

- Bacterial infection

Increased eosinophils may indicate:

- Allergy
- Parasitic infection
- Asthma

Increased lymphocytes may indicate:

- Infectious mononucleosis

Platelet Count

Platelets are non-nucleated cells formed in the bone marrow from a large parent cell called the megakaryocyte. They play an important role in the coagulation cascade and in vasoconstriction.

Normal: 140–415 × 10E3/uL (140,000–400,000 mm^3)

If there is a marked decrease, <20,000, there is a risk of spontaneous bleeding.

Thrombocytopenia may indicate

- Idiopathic thrombocytopenic purpura
- Bone marrow pathologies
- Alcohol abuse

Increased platelets may indicate:

- Leukemia
- Polycythemia vera
- Splenectomy
- Hodgkin's disease

Managing Hypocoagulability

If a patient comes in with an increased tendency to bleed or bruise, the following tests should be done:

- Prothrombin time (PT)
- Partial thromboplastin time (PTT)
- Platelet count

ILLUSTRATIVE CASE FOR PRACTICE

A 52-year-old white female came in with the chief complaints of:

- Tiredness
- Shortness of breath (SOB) upon exertion

Duration of symptoms: Six months.

Past history (PH): Gravida two; parity two; hysterectomy five years ago.

Physical exam (PE): Vitals normal, except pulse, which was 110 bpm.

Additional PE: Premature gray hair and pallor in the conjunctiva and skin.

Question 1 Suspecting that her symptoms may be caused by anemia and you are also concerned about her SOB, what test would you order first?

A. CBC.

B. Troponin.

C. Chest X-ray.

D. Electrocardiogram.

The correct response is A.

Clinically, she appears anemic. This would also explain her complaints, so this should be investigated first. The results of her CBC are as follows (ranges are listed in the final column):

WBC	4.8 × 10E3/uL	4.0–10.5
RBC	3.91 × 10E6/uL	3.80–5.10
Hemoglobin	9.7 g/dL (low)	11.5–15.0
Hematocrit	37.6%	34.0–44.0
MCV	105 fL (high)	80–98
MCH	32.5 pg	27.0–34.0
MCHC	33.8 g/dL	32.0–36.0
RDW	14.0%	11.7–15.0
Platelets	220 × 10E3/uL	140–415
Neutrophils	52%	40–74
Lymphocytes	38%	14–46
Monocytes	7%	4–13
Eosophils	2%	0–7
Neutrophils (absolute)	2.5 × 10E3/uL	1.8–7.8
Lymphocytes (absolute)	1.8 × 10E3/uL	0.7–4.5
Monocytes (absolute)	0.3 × 10E3/uL	0.1–1.0
Eosophils (absolute)	0.1 × 10E3/uL	0.0–0.4
Basophils (absolute)	0.0 × 10E3/uL	0.0–0.2
Immature granulocytes	0%	0–1
Immature granulocytes (absolute)	0.0 × 10E3/uL	0.0–0.1

Abbreviations: MCH, mean corpuscular hemoglobin; MCHC, mean cell hemoglobin concentration; MCV, mean corpuscular volume; RBC, red blood cell; RDW, red cell distribution width; WBC, white blood cell.

Question 2 What is your conclusion after reading the CBC?

A. She is anemic.

B. She is not anemic.

C. Her SOB is probably related to a cardiac or pulmonary cause.

D. This is a menopausal problem.

The correct response is A.

Her hemoglobin should have been 11.5 g/dL but is only 9.7 g/dL.

Question 3 What should we look at next, and what conclusion can we make?

A. Look at the MCV. She has microcytic anemia.

B. Look at the MCV. She has macrocytic anemia.

C. Look at the MCV. She has normocytic anemia.

D. As the patient is symptomatic of anemia, she should be treated with an iron supplement.

The correct response is B.

As her MCV is 105, she has macrocytic anemia.

Response D shows poor judgment; treatment with an iron supplement should never be the next step.

Question 4 What conclusions can you make from the information provided so far?

A. Patient has either folic acid or vitamin B12 deficiency.

B. Patient has iron deficiency.

C. Patient has hemolytic anemia.

D. There is a problem with her bone marrow.

The correct response is A.

The two etiologies of macrocytic anemia are either vitamin B12 deficiency or folic acid deficiency.

Question 5 What should be the next step?

A. Perform second-line blood test to find the exact cause of her macrocytic anemia (i.e., check vitamin B12 level and folic acid level).

B. Start treatment with vitamin B12 replacement.

C. Perform a bone marrow aspiration.

D. Get a cardiac consultation.

The correct response is A.

Results from testing reveal a very low vitamin B12 level.

Question 6 What other features are often seen in a peripheral blood smear obtained from a person with vitamin B12 deficiency?

A. Reticulocytosis.

B. Increased number of hypersegmented polymorphs.

C. Tear drop cells.

D. Increased platelets.

The correct response is B.

Question 7 What is the other name for macrocytic anemia?

A. Megaloblastic anemia.

B. Aplastic anemia.

C. Anemia of chronic illness.

D. Sideroblastic anemia.

The correct response is A.

The statistical likelihood is that this patient suffers from an auto-immune disease that is destroying the cells of the stomach that produce intrinsic factor. Without intrinsic factor, vitamin B12 cannot be absorbed; this is also known as pernicious anemia. Treatment with active vitamin B12 (methylcolbalamin) should be started, preferably as an intramuscular (IM) injection.

Question 8 This action (treating with vitamin B12) shows:

A. Poor judgment. Further studies should be done and no treatment decisions made on statistics.

B. Good judgment. This is the recommended practice as further checking would only delay treatment.

C. Good judgment. Start oral vitamin B12 replacement.

D. Start vitamin B12 and iron together.

The correct response is B.

The most common cause of vitamin B12 deficiency is auto-immune destruction of intrinsic factor producing stomach cells, which is necessary for vitamin B12 absorption.

Question 9 The replacement should be done by:

A. Oral replacement.

B. IM injection.

C. Sublingual replacement.

D. Intravenous (IV).

The correct response is B.

Without intrinsic factor, B12 will not be absorbed at its usual place of absorption (ileum), therefore an oral administration would be ineffective.

TCM PERSPECTIVE

This patient may present with a thin or thread-like pulse and a pale, dry tongue. Upon making a diagnosis of blood deficiency per TCM, best practice would be to order a CBC or request one from the patient's primary care physician (PCP). Tonifying acupuncture treatments and blood nourishing herbs may indeed help address this patient's complaints, but the patient will not experience complete symptom resolution until vitamin B12 levels are adequately restored. Therefore, an integrated approach would be to include a CBC when you suspect a blood deficiency. It is also useful and considered best practice to order a CBC when infection is suspected or the complaint is of unexplained fatigue. Remember, an integrated approach relies upon the fact that you as a professional will refer out to the appropriate specialist or, at a minimum, to the PCP, when seriously abnormal results are found.

2

HEMOCCULT

BASIC SCIENCE

Treating a patient with iron replacement, immediately after a diagnosis of anemia or iron-deficiency anemia is made, can be dangerous. An etiology for the anemia should always be sought first. For example, the GI tract is often the site of the blood loss in people with iron-deficiency anemia. Therefore, if the site of bleeding is not obvious, the stool should be checked for blood. If the stool test for blood is positive, the exact site of the problem can be found subsequently by endoscopy or by radiological studies.

HEMOCCULT TEST

The hemoccult, which is a cardboard square with an incorporated test strip, is given to the patient. The patient takes it home and, at the time of his/her next bowel movement, smears a stool sample on the hemoccult. The hemoccult is brought back to the office, where it is tested with a developer. If blood is present, a blue color develops. As the test is very sensitive, one should be mindful about false positives and false negatives.

TCM PERSPECTIVE

If, as a TCM practitioner, you suspect that a patient has bleeding from the GI system (not obvious bleeding from a hemorrhoid or anal fissure), then the appropriate and best practice action is referral to the PCP. This does not mean you must stop your treatment.

3

THE KIDNEYS AND THE
URINARY SYSTEM

BASIC SCIENCE
Kidney Functions

- Excrete nitrogenous wastes—primary function
- Maintain water balance
- Maintain electrolyte balance
- Maintain pH balance
- Perform endocrine functions, which include secreting:
  - renin
  - 1,25 vitamin D

- ○ erythropoietin
- Maintain blood pressure

These kidney functions are maintained by an adequate flow of blood through the kidney at all times. The rate at which blood is cleaned in the kidneys is called glomerular filtration rate (GFR), which normally is 120 ml/min. At the time of protein metabolism, the nitrogen is converted into ammonia, a toxic substance for the body. This ammonia is converted by the liver to a less noxious substance called blood urea nitrogen (BUN). The kidney excretes BUN along with creatinine, which is formed by the breakdown of muscle cells and uric acid. Of the endocrine functions, erythropoietin stimulates the bone marrow to form RBCs. Renin, along with other subsequent endocrine secretions, helps maintain volume and blood pressure, whereas 1,25 vitamin D helps calcium and bone metabolism and has many other protective roles. The nephron, or the functional kidney unit, makes an ultra-infiltrate of the blood at the glomerulus. Most of the essential substances are reabsorbed at the proximal convoluted tubule. At the loop of Henle, a variable percentage of water and electrolytes are reabsorbed depending on the needs of the body. Other substances such as potassium, hydrogen, and creatinine are also added to the urine by secretion into the nephron at the convoluted tubules. All of the above results in the excretion of about 1500 cc of urine every day. Normal urine should not contain any blood cells or protein, as they are never filtered (except very small amounts of protein, usually not detected by standard tests). Whenever there is impairment of the kidney function there is a simultaneous decrease in GFR, even before blood tests show any change. This makes GFR an excellent measure of kidney function.

BLOOD TESTS FOR KIDNEY FUNCTION

A common way to assess kidney function is to measure the concentration of substances the kidney usually excretes:

BUN

Normal: 6–20 mg/dL

Creatinine

Normal: 0.6–1.2 mg/dL

Any increase in these values suggests impairment of kidney function. BUN might be falsely elevated due to:

- Dehydration
- Bleeding in the GI tract

Very commonly, at the time of kidney failure, potassium values increase. Therefore, when BUN and creatinine are elevated, potassium values also should be assessed (and addressed if abnormal), as the safety window is very small.

Potassium

Normal: 3.5–5.5 mmol/L

With worsening of the kidney function, a few additional changes may be noted:

- Acidosis, as shown by decreased bicarbonate
- Increase of uric acid due to impaired excretion
- Decrease in calcium due to decrease of 1,25 vitamin D
- Anemia due to decrease in erythropoietin

In summary, abnormal blood values seen in kidney failure are:

- BUN—increased
- Creatinine—increased

- Potassium—increased
- Bicarbonate—decreased
- Uric acid—increased
- Calcium—decreased
- Anemia may be present as shown by a decrease in hemoglobin

However, as the kidney has tremendous reserve, the above tests do not show changes until about 60% of the kidney function is decreased. Therefore, it is best to order tests that will measure GFR in order to identify early renal impairment.

Tests to Determine GFR

In the past, inulin was injected into a person and the GFR was determined from the rate of excretion. A later discovery found that GFR could be calculated by measuring creatinine in the urine and in the blood. The test was called creatinine clearance. Today, creatinine clearance is still considered an excellent early test; however, instead of doing a timed urine collection and blood test, creatinine clearance can be calculated using the serum creatinine value. A decrease in GFR is the earliest sign of kidney disease, especially in patients with diabetes mellitus, and GFR should be tested annually so that therapeutic changes can be made.

Urinalysis

Urine checking is also an important diagnostic tool. In the past, urinalysis was done in the laboratory, but now most of the tests can be done in the office using chemically impregnated strips called dipsticks. Results are obtained by observing the color change and matching it with the original color of the dipstick as depicted on the side of the container. Microscopic analysis of the urine provides additional information that the dipstick is incapable of producing; however, it is recommended that a dipstick analysis be done initially.

The dipstick assessment gives information about the following:

- Specific gravity
- pH
- Glucose
- Blood
- Bilirubin
- Urobilinogen
- Protein
- Nitrite
- Leucocytes
- Ketones

Note: The presence of glucose does not confirm a diagnosis of diabetes. The presence of ketones in the absence of glycosuria suggests that the patient has been in a starved state versus a well-fed state. The presence of ketones along with high urinary glucose raises the possibility of diabetic ketoacidosis. The presence of bilirubin and urobilinogen suggests liver disease. The specific gravity tells us about the hydration status of the patient and the capability of the kidney to concentrate urine.

Assessment should be done at the precise time suggested. The usual diagnoses by dipstick include:

- Urinary tract infection (UTI). This is suggested whenever there is presence of leucocytes or nitrites.

Presence of blood and proteins is suggestive of infection but not confirmatory.

• Hematuria—presence of blood in the urine.

• Proteinuria—presence of protein in the urine (see below).

It is advisable for all practitioners to have and use dipstick urinalysis in their clinics. However, there will be occasions, although rare, when a microscopic examination will be necessary.

Examination of the centrifuged urine sediment may add the following information:

• The presence of casts suggests that the pathology is present in the kidney and not in the urinary bladder. The type of cast also helps in making some diagnosis.

• The presence of crystals suggests high uric acid and higher risks for urinary stones.

• Microscopic examination will also reconfirm the presence or absence of leukocytes and RBCs that were noted on dipstick examination.

Proteinuria

The degree of proteinuria has great diagnostic significance. If the dipstick shows that a large amount of protein is present, a 24-hour urine collection for quantitative measurement of protein should be done. Further diagnosis, such as nephrotic syndrome, may be made based on the amount of protein present.

WHAT IS NEPHROTIC SYNDROME?

In many diseases of the kidney, as the kidney function worsens, more and more protein is excreted in the urine.

The criterion for nephrotic syndrome is excretion of >3.5 g of protein in 24 hours. This leads to hypoproteinemia with the resultant low oncotic pressure leading to edema and hyperlipidemia.

ILLUSTRATIVE CASE FOR PRACTICE

This 38-year-old man was seen at the clinic for severe right-sided low back pain of one day duration. The pain starts in the back and radiates down to his groin. His urine has an unusual dark color. He does not remember injuring his back or lifting anything heavy in the last week. He has been feeling tired for the last six months and has been taking energy tonics and vitamin B12 injections.

PH: Nothing significant.

Family history (FH): Father had prostate cancer.

Social history (SH): Patient smokes a pack of 20 cigarettes per 24 hours.

PE: A well-nourished young male (with BMI of 23), who appears to be in moderate distress. Rest of the PE was within normal limits, except for low back pain and tenderness.

Vitals: Blood pressure 140/90 mmHg.

Question 1 What are your differential diagnoses?

A. Muscular pain.

B. Urinary tract problem, kidney stone or infection.

C. Joint pain involving the spine.

D. Acute pancreatitis.

The correct response is B.

Musculoskeletal pain (A) is also possible and should remain a part of the thought process.

D is very unlikely as this is a very unusual presentation for acute pancreatitis.

Question 2 What would you do next?

A. Do a dipstick assessment of his urine at the clinic.

B. Send him to get a CBC and chemistry profile.

C. Prescribe some analgesics and have him return in a week.

D. Refer him to an orthopedic surgeon.

The correct response is A.

A urinary tract problem appears to be the most likely cause. Urinary tract infection in a 38-year-old male without obstruction is very unlikely. If the urine analysis comes back as normal, the likelihood of it being simple musculoskeletal pain increases. At this stage, an orthopedic surgical consultation would be inappropriate and cause the patient unnecessary expense.

The dipstick urine analysis showed the following:

1. Specific gravity: 1005

2. Occult blood: 4+

3. WBC: (-) negative

4. Nitrite: (-)

5. Glucose: (-)

6. Ketone: (-)

7. Bilirubin: (-)

Question 3 What is your conclusion from the urine analysis results?

A. UTI.

B. Diabetes mellitus.

C. Hematuria.

D. Normal urine.

The correct response is C.

Question 4 What is the most likely diagnosis?

A. Cancer of the kidney.

B. Kidney stones.

C. Pyelonephritis.

D. Trauma.

The correct response is B.

If there is blood in his urine in conjunction with severe low back pain, he most likely has a kidney stone.

The patient was sent to the emergency room (ER) because of the severe back pain. He was treated with pain medication and imaging was ordered. The computerized tomography (CT) scan showed two very small stones in his left ureter with no other abnormality apparent. With relaxation from the pain medication and higher volume intravenous fluids the patient eventually passed both stones. The patient was released from the ER and has returned to see you on the next day. He does not have any more pain, but is tired from his day at the ER and the pain medication. His repeat urine dipstick test is completely normal.

Question 5 What is the next step?

A. Nothing further needs to be done as he is pain-free and has passed his stones.

B. Further investigation needs to be done or else he may have kidney stones in the future.

C. He may have uric acid stones.

D. He may have triple phosphate stones.

The correct response is B.

Though some authorities believe that one episode of kidney stone does not call for further investigation, opinion is divided. It is often best to ask the patient for their opinion. Most patients would prefer to avoid future events and pain.

Question 6 What are the different kinds of kidney stone?

A. Calcium.

B. Uric acid.

C. Triple phosphate (struvite).

D. All of the above.

The correct response is D.

Calcium stones are by far the most common (80%). Uric acid stones are usually associated with elevated uric acid and gout. Triple phosphate stones are much more common in females and are usually associated with repeated UTIs.

The patient was asked to drink large amounts of fluid and prepare for additional tests.

Question 7 What tests would you order next?

A. Chemistry profile.

B. Urine analysis.

C. Urine culture.

D. This is too complicated and patient should be referred out.

The correct response is A.

This would determine high calcium or high uric acid. Further examination of the urine will not help. The results of the chemistry profile were as follows (ranges are listed in the final column):

CBC with Differential/Platelet

WBC	3.0 × 10E3/uL	4.0–10.5
RBC	4.64 × 10E6/uL	3.80–5.10
Hemoglobin	14.3 g/dL	11.5–15.0
Hematocrit	40.4%	34.0–44.0
MCV	87 fL	80–98
MCH	30.7 pg	27.0–34.0
MCHC	35.3 g/dL	32.0–36.0
RDW	13.1%	11.7–15.0
Platelets	277 × 10E3/uL	140–415
Neutrophils	45%	40–74
Lymphocytes	37%	14–46
Monocytes	13%	4–13
Eosophils	4%	0–7
Basophils	1%	0–3
Neutrophils (absolute)	1.4 × 10E3/uL (low)	1.8–7.8
Lymphocytes (absolute)	1.1 × 10E3/uL	0.7–4.5
Monocytes (absolute)	0.4 × 10E3/uL	0.1–1.0
Eosophils (absolute)	0.1 × 10E3/uL	0.0–0.4
Basophils (absolute)	0.0 × 10E3/uL	0.0–0.2

Basic Metabolic Panel

Glucose, serum	82 mg/dL	65–99
BUN	13 mg/dL	5–26
Creatinine, serum	0.8 mg/dL	0.57–1.00
BUN/creatinine ratio	16 mg/dL	8–27
Sodium, serum	138 mmol/L	135–144
Potassium, serum	3.8 mmol/L	3.5–5.2
Chloride, serum	103 mmol/L	96–108
Carbon dioxide, total	25 mmol/L	20–32
Calcium, serum	11.0 mg/dL (high)	8.6–10.2

Abbreviations: BUN, blood urea nitrogen; CBC, complete blood count; MCH, mean corpuscular hemoglobin; MCHC, mean cell hemoglobin concentration; MCV, mean corpuscular volume; RBC, red blood cell; RDW, red cell distribution width; WBC, white blood cell.

Question 8 After you look at the above results, what is the next test that you should order?

A. Bone scan.

B. Parathyroid hormone level.

C. Refer to a rheumatologist for joint aspiration.

D. No further testing is required.

The correct response is B.

This is indicated due to elevated calcium.
    Parathyroid hormone level comes back elevated.

Question 9 What is your conclusion?

A. Hyperparathyroidism.

B. Gout.

C. Ask the patient or decrease his calcium intake.

D. Not enough information to make any further conclusions.

The correct response is A.

This patient should be referred to an endocrinologist for management of his hyperparathyroidism.

TCM PERSPECTIVE

In my experience, TCM practitioners seem to shy away from ordering or requesting studies for their patients. As you gain knowledge and utilize laboratory testing in the clinic/classroom, confidence will develop and it will serve to benefit your patients and your treatment outcomes. It is my opinion that using a urine analysis test would provide the evidence base to support treatment of UTIs and other disorders of the urinary system with Oriental medicine modalities and techniques. We must take advantage of the diagnostic capabilities conventional science affords us. In this way, we are sure of what we are treating and we can justify why we took a particular course of action. Evidence-based testing supports the direction of our treatment plans and provides us with baselines to prove outcomes and efficacy of treatment.

4

WATER, ELECTROLYTES, AND PH BALANCE

This chapter covers material more commonly seen within an "in-patient" setting than in TCM outpatient practice. With that in mind, the subject is not covered extensively, and interested practitioners may have to refer to standard textbooks. Water constitutes 60% of the human body, with approximately two-thirds of it being intracellular and one-third extracellular. The human body does not tolerate fluid deficit or excess well, if at all. If any of these abnormalities are present, they must be quickly identified and corrected.

Though there are many clinical features of volume-related complications, there are only a few laboratory tests that are helpful.

ELECTROLYTES

The electrolytes discussed in this chapter are:

- Sodium
- Potassium
- Calcium
- Magnesium

Sodium

Sodium is the most abundant extra cellular electrolyte, and serum levels are assessed to identify volume complications more than any other test.

Serum sodium

Normal: 135–144 mmol/L

Etiology of hypernatremia:

- Volume depletion
- Mineral corticoid excess

The most common cause of hypernatremia is volume depletion. Clinically, an additional confirmation can be made by assessing for orthostatic hypotension. Depending on the severity of volume depletion, the clinical state may be dangerous, as it may result in decreased blood supply to the brain, reduced cardiac output and a reduction in GFR.

Etiology of hyponatremia:

- Pseudohyponatremia
- Hyperosmolar hyponatremia
- Hypovolemic hyponatremia

- Syndrome of inappropriate antidiuretic hormone (SIADH)
- Addison's disease

Potassium

Potassium is the most abundant intracellular electrolyte, and maintaining a safe range is critical as it is very narrow. Levels that drop <3 mmol/L or rise >6 mmol/L can be dangerous, as this may lead to cardiac arrhythmia or severe muscle weakness.

Serum potassium

Normal: 3.5–5.2 mmol/L

Etiology of hyperkalemia:

- Renal failure
- Pseudohyperkalemia
- Drugs (e.g., angiotensin-converting-enzyme inhibitor (ACE) inhibitors, potassium-sparing diuretics)

Etiology of hypokalemia:

- Diuretics
- GI loss
- Hyperaldosteronism

Calcium

Serum calcium

Normal: 8.6–10.2 mg/dL

Approximately 50% of circulating calcium in the blood is free or ionized, the rest is protein bound to albumin with the majority of storage in the bone. If calcium levels fall too low, serious problems, such as laryngospasm or cardiac issues may result.

Etiology of hypercalcemia:

- Hyperparathyroidism

- Malignancy (seen in paraneoplastic syndrome and in metastatic bone disease)

- Hypervitaminosis D

Etiology of hypocalcemia:

- Hypoparathyroidism

- Vitamin D deficiency

- Pseudohypocalcemia

Magnesium

Serum magnesium

Normal: 1.5–2.3 mg/dL

Etiology of hypermagnesemia:

- Renal failure

- Addison's disease

- Excessive intake of magnesium as a supplement

Etiology of hypomagnesemia:

- Malabsorption

- Drugs

- Chronic alcoholism

Acid-Base Imbalance

The pH of the blood is maintained at 7.35–7.45, and it is tightly regulated at this level for normal cellular functioning. If the level changes, it is quickly corrected by mechanisms that include carbonic acid–bicarbonate, protein and phosphate buffering systems. Organs of importance in these systems are the lung and kidney, both utilized to buffer the acid–base balance by the functions of exhaling carbon dioxide and the elimination of hydrogen via the kidneys.

pH

Normal: 7.35–7.45

The four complications that are seen with acid–base problems are:

1. Metabolic acidosis

2. Metabolic alkalosis

3. Respiratory acidosis

4. Respiratory alkalosis

These may occur singularly or in combination.

The best test to detect a change in pH is an arterial blood gas, but as this is not usually performed in an outpatient setting by TCM practitioners, we will not discuss it here. The majority of patients suffering from one of these complications will most likely already be in critical care.

ILLUSTRATIVE CASE FOR PRACTICE

This 16-year-old white male was brought to the ER after having passed out while playing basketball with his friends on a hot summer afternoon.

History of Present Illness (HPI): Patient has been in good health all his life.

PH: None.

FH: Father has high blood pressure.

SH: Patient does not smoke or drink.

Review of systems: Within normal limits (WNL).

PE: A well-nourished young male (with BMI of 23), who appears to be in moderate distress. Rest of the physical examination was entirely normal except for signs of volume depletion.

Vitals: Blood pressure 120/70 mmHg while supine, and 90/60 mmHg while standing.

The assumption is that the patient had a syncopal episode due to dehydration and heat exposure. The drop in orthostatic blood pressure also suggested dehydration. An electrolyte panel blood test was drawn and patient was started on high volume saline solution IV. He was also encouraged to drink fluids.

The test results showed that his serum sodium levels were 150 mmol/L, confirming the diagnosis of hypovolemia.

TCM PERSPECTIVE

Although it is good to understand these tests in order to treat patients post-incident, more than likely we would not see hypovolemia in a private practice setting. However, this would be excellent information to have when you are creating a treatment plan to prevent future episodes. In my opinion, there are many misconceptions around the acid balance topic in holistic healthcare. It is a complex biochemical topic, which means most lay people do not understand the body's natural buffering mechanisms and how little acute change food and drink can make. It is our responsibility, as integrated practitioners, to assist our patents in understanding basic biochemical facts related to pH balance. In the long-term, a balanced diet that has less stress on the buffering systems will benefit patients much more than utilizing alkaline water, for instance, to make an immediate change.

5

GLUCOSE METABOLISM
AND DIABETES
MELLITUS

BASIC SCIENCE

The human body maintains glucose levels between 80–110 mg/dL. This ensures that enough glucose is available as a ready source of energy. Glucose levels are maintained from food intake in a postprandial state, from liver glycogen stored when not eating, and by conversion from amino acids during starvation. The brain's sole source of energy is glucose and its function is impaired if the level drops below 40 mg/dL. If the level of glucose exceeds normal, insulin is secreted to drive the glucose into the cell for immediate use and future storage. If it gets too high, >180 mg/dL, the body will excrete the excess glucose in the urine in an additional effort to lower levels to normal. If the level of glucose gets too low, hormones such as glucagon, cortisol, and growth hormone will help raise it.

Diabetes Mellitus

Diabetes mellitus is a heterogeneous group of metabolic diseases characterized by hyperglycemia due to impaired secretion or function of insulin.

There are different types of diabetes mellitus:

- Type 1
- Type 2
- Gestational

MANAGEMENT OF DIABETES MELLITUS

With diet, exercise, and medical management, the glucose level must be kept as close to normal as possible, without lowering it to a hypoglycemic state. If the glucose level gets too high or too low, acute complications may result.

Acute Complications of Diabetes Mellitus

- Diabetic ketoacidosis
- Hyperosmolar non-ketotic diabetic coma
- Hypoglycemia

Even moderate elevations of blood glucose over a period of years could lead to chronic complications.

Chronic Complications of Diabetes Mellitus

- Retinopathy, often leading to blindness
- Cardiac issues
- Renal impairment, often requiring dialysis
- Non-traumatic amputation of the lower limb

Gestational Diabetes Mellitus

The danger of moderate hyperglycemia becomes even more serious in gestational diabetes mellitus. It is my opinion that glucose levels should be kept under 100 mg/dL at all times. If it is not, both the baby and the mother may be injured, and the outcome of pregnancy will be less than desirable.

Blood Tests for Diabetes Mellitus

BLOOD GLUCOSE

When assessing blood glucose, the following points should be considered:

1. Fasting blood glucose

    Normal: 70–110 mg/dL

    This is the most useful test and it must be performed after a 12-hour fast.

2. Random blood glucose

    In this test, the blood glucose level is checked with no consideration as to when the last meal was consumed.

3. Postprandial blood glucose—2 hour

    Normal: <140 mg dl/L

The blood glucose level is checked two hours after a substantial meal. This is a modified glucose stress test, challenging the system's metabolic capabilities after a somewhat regular meal.

4. Glucose tolerance test

The blood glucose level is checked at periodic intervals after ingesting a high load of glucose. This test is not utilized as extensively now, except for a modified version used in the diagnosis of gestational diabetes mellitus.

5. Glycated hemoglobin (HbA1c)

Normal: <5.7% (39 mmol/mol)

Diabetes: 6.5% (47 mmol/mol) and above

Risk of developing diabetes in the future: 5.7–6.4% (39–46 mmol/mol)

This test allows for an observation of the varying ranges of glucose over the preceding 90 days. With this information we can make assumptions as to how the patient is controlling their diet or how well the treatment plan is working.

6. Glutamic acid decarboxylase (GAD) and islet cell auto-antibodies (ICA) are markers of auto-immune destruction of the beta cells of the pancreas and are often seen in type 1 diabetes mellitus.

Urine Tests for Diabetes Mellitus
GLUCOSE

Detection of glucose in the urine is not very helpful in the care of patients with diabetes mellitus; if glucose is present, it usually suggests poor control.

Presence of glucose in the urine of a patient who is not known to be diabetic calls for an evaluation of a fasting blood glucose.

Test to Monitor Kidney Function in Diabetes Mellitus

MICROALBUMIN

Presence of microalbumin in the urine may be the earliest sign of diabetic nephropathy. All diabetic patients' urine should be checked at least once a year for microalbumin. Once microalbumin is detected, blood kidney function tests and quantitative protein measurement in urine should be done at regular intervals.

QUANTITATIVE PROTEIN

When kidney function declines, the amount of protein excreted in the urine gradually increases. Initially, there is no protein; next, upon worsening function, microalbumin is detected, and then finally, a trace amount of protein can be detected. With worsening conditions, >1 of protein may be excreted in 24 hours and finally the result will be overt nephrotic syndrome.

In order to monitor kidney function, standard blood tests should be done at regular intervals in people with diabetes mellitus. These include the following:

- BUN

- Creatinine

- Electrolytes

It is important to note, again, that because the kidney has tremendous reserves, abnormalities do not show up in standard kidney function tests until very late. Creatinine clearance should be done at regular intervals because of this. Though this is an excellent test, it is more difficult to do because it entails a 24-hour urine collection and a simultaneous blood test. Serum creatinine is used to calculate the GFR using the Cockcroft–Gault formula because of these difficulties. Even without using the formula, the serum creatinine does give a rough estimate of the GFR.

- When serum creatinine is normal (0.57–1.00), GFR is also normal (120 mL/min).

- When serum creatinine is increased to 2, GFR is decreased to 60 mL/min.

- Unfortunately, with further increase in serum creatinine, this simple linear relation is lost, and by the time the serum creatinine is 4, GFR is <20 mL/min.

Keep the following in mind when seeking answers for these four common questions related to diabetes mellitus:

QUESTION 1: DOES THE PATIENT HAVE DIABETES MELLITUS?

A diagnosis of diabetes mellitus can be made in the following circumstances:

- Fasting blood glucose is >126 mg/dL (with a minimum of two separate date/time readings).

- Clinical features of diabetes mellitus are apparent.

- Random blood glucose is >200 mg/dL.

- Glycated hemoglobin (HbA1c), however, should not be used to make a diagnosis of diabetes mellitus.

Note: Different criteria are used for the diagnosis of gestational diabetes mellitus, and any patient fitting these criteria should be referred out immediately.

QUESTION 2: WHAT KIND OF DIABETES MELLITUS DOES THE PATIENT HAVE?

- Type 1 diabetes mellitus is more commonly seen in the young. They are underweight and have had clinical features of diabetes mellitus for a short time, usually days.

- Type 2 diabetes mellitus is more commonly seen in overweight adults who may have had some features of diabetes mellitus for months or years.

Specific Testing for Type 1 Diabetes Mellitus

Serum insulin or C-peptide is often absent; however, these tests are not always accurate. The most definitive test for diabetes mellitus type I measures the presence of Islet cell antibodies or GAD.

QUESTION 3: HOW WELL IS THE PATIENT'S DIABETES MELLITUS CONTROLLED?

- Abnormal blood glucose levels can lead to acute and chronic complications; therefore, glucose levels have to be kept as close to normal as possible.

- To ascertain chronic blood glucose levels, repeated blood glucose testing needs to be checked and recorded by the patient with home blood glucose monitoring. Both fasting and postprandial blood glucose should be checked often. Checking should not be limited to the morning only but done at different times on different days.

- HbA1c should be checked three or four times a year and, ideally, kept between 6.5% and 7.0%.

QUESTION 4: DOES THE PATIENT HAVE ANY COMPLICATIONS OF DIABETES MELLITUS?

The chances that a TCM practitioner or student will encounter acute complications of diabetes mellitus, such as diabetic ketoacidosis, are small; however, seeing a patient with hypoglycemia is not unusual.

Hypoglycemia

Though a diabetic patient may be confused, comatose, or obtunded from various etiologies, it is imperative that hypoglycemia is always ruled out first. Blood glucose level can be obtained adequately by a finger stick, for which any home glucose monitoring device will suffice. Blood glucose <50 mg/dL should be considered as hypoglycemia and treated promptly. Please remember that it is very dangerous to give anything by mouth to an unconscious patient.

Diabetic Ketoacidosis

This is usually observed in type 1 diabetes mellitus but may also occur in type 2 diabetes mellitus. It is usually caused by an absolute or relative lack of insulin. The two common situations for which patients are often brought in with ketoacidosis are infections and missed insulin injections. The patient presents with confusion or coma, is usually hyperventilating from acidosis, is severely dehydrated and has breath that may smell of acetone, which smells like Juicy Fruit gum. This patient, if encountered in a private practice setting must be referred for emergency care immediately.

Laboratory abnormalities in diabetic ketoacidosis are found in:

- Urine
  - Ketones are elevated
  - Glucose is elevated
- Blood
  - Glucose is elevated
  - Bicarbonate is decreased
  - Potassium is abnormal

  Despite total body potassium being low due to the acidosis, there is always a transcellular shift. As a result, serum potassium may initially be elevated, but as the acidosis is corrected, there will be sudden drop in potassium level.

Diabetic ketoacidosis is a dire medical emergency and the patient must be sent immediately for emergency care.

Detection of Chronic Complications of Diabetes Mellitus

Most chronic complications of diabetes mellitus (retinopathy, cardiovascular problems, and neuropathy) are usually detected clinically rather than by laboratory testing. The exception is diabetic nephropathy, where laboratory testing is very helpful. After a person has been diabetic for a few years, especially if blood glucose and blood pressure are not adequately controlled, kidney damage will occur. Initially, there is hyperperfusion of the kidneys and soon afterwards, there will be a gradual decrease in glomerular filtration rate. An early marker of kidney damage is the presence of microalbumin in the urine. With further worsening of the kidney function, the amount of protein in the urine will increase until the patient is in overt nephrotic syndrome. It is important, in the care of patients with diabetes, to perform kidney function testing regularly, so that early evidence of kidney dysfunction is detected and treated.

ILLUSTRATIVE CASE FOR PRACTICE

A 50-year-old male came in with the complaints of polyuria and polydipsia. He also complained of some blurring of his vision and a metallic taste in his mouth. The problems had probably been going on for the last three or four months.

PH: Hernia surgery ten years ago.

FH: Mother has diabetes mellitus.

SH: Patient does not smoke. Patient drinks beer occasionally.

Review of systems: Unremarkable.

PE: BMI = 30. Vital signs normal. Physical examination is WNL.

Question 1 As many of his features suggest diabetes mellitus, how is the diagnosis of diabetes mellitus made?

A. Check urine for glucose.

B. Check HbA1c.

C. Check fasting blood glucose, preferably more than one time.

D. Perform a glucose tolerance test.

The correct response is C.

A diagnosis of diabetes mellitus is made by checking fasting blood glucose; if the fasting blood glucose level is >126 mg/dL, diabetes is indicated.

Question 2 Though this person might appear to have type 2 diabetes, what test(s) can be done to rule out type 1?

A. Type 1 is only present in children.

B. Patients with type 1 are always underweight.

C. Measure GAD and islet cell antibodies.

D. Measure C-peptide.

The correct response is C.

A, B, and D may apply to type 1; but the best response is C.

The patient's fasting blood glucose on two occasions was >300 mg/dL. A diagnosis of diabetes was made.

Question 3 What are some of the presenting features that would make you suspect diabetes?

A. Polyuria and polydipsia.

B. Blurring of vision.

C. Chronic yeast infections.

D. All of the above.

The correct response is D.

The above features in all patients should result in an evaluation for diabetes mellitus. A strong family history of diabetes mellitus in conjunction with high birth weight infants (greater than 10 pounds) should also be a reason to check for diabetes mellitus.

Question 4 What are the chronic complications of diabetes mellitus?

A. Heart disease.

B. Kidney failure.

C. Blindness.

D. All of the above.

The correct response is D.

In addition to the above, non-traumatic amputation of the leg is another chronic complication of diabetes mellitus. This is explained in detail to the patient. He is reminded again that if he neglects proper care of the diabetes and allows his blood glucose to run high, it is just a matter of time before the chronic complications appear. Proper care of diabetes mellitus requires periodic checking of his blood glucose control and monitoring his opthalmic, kidney, cardiovascular, and neurologic systems.

Question 5 Other than self/home blood glucose checking, how else can a practitioner monitor the control of glucose levels?

A. Measuring glucose in 24-hour urine.

B. Checking HbA1c.

C. Checking blood glucose at each clinic visit.

D. Checking for complications.

The correct response is B.

According to the American Diabetes Association, HbA1c should ideally be maintained at <7%. HbA1c should be checked three to four times a year in addition to the regular home blood glucose checking.

Question 6 What tests should be done to closely monitor kidney functions?

A. BUN and creatinine should be checked in blood.

B. Microalbumin should be checked.

C. CT scan of the kidney.

D. A kidney biopsy.

The correct response is B.

Microalbumin and creatinine clearance should be checked once or twice every year.

TCM PERSPECTIVE

Understanding laboratory testing for diabetes is essential in monitoring your patient's progress with TCM treatment. Most diabetic patients are very savvy and utilize conventional language to discuss their health concerns. Most request help from TCM practitioners with controlling their blood glucose levels and weight loss. Ordering and following their laboratory results makes you a more professional, thorough, and credible practitioner. In addition, with so many TCM protocols, having a baseline laboratory report can further provide evidence to the PCP or endocrinologist that your treatment strategies are indeed effective.

6

LIVER FUNCTION

BASIC SCIENCE

Liver Functions

- Detoxification of exogenous and endogenous substances.

- Synthesis of many important proteins.

- Synthesis and storage of many important metabolites, including glucose.

- Production and excretion of bile.

Bilirubin Metabolism

Most of the bilirubin comes from the breakdown of aging RBCs by the reticuloendothelial (RE) system. The liver removes the bilirubin from the blood and excretes it in the bile. There are two forms of bilirubin:

1. Unconjugated bilirubin: Unconjugated bilirubin, also known as indirect bilirubin, is made in the RE system, is insoluble and carried as a protein bound form to the liver. There it is conjugated with glucoronic acid, and thus becomes soluble, and is then excreted in the bile.

2. Conjugated bilirubin: Conjugated bilirubin, also known as direct bilirubin, is the form of bilirubin after being conjugated with glucoronic acid. Once this form of bilirubin enters the intestine, it is converted to urobilinogen, which is mostly excreted in the feces. About 20% of urobilinogen is reabsorbed and then excreted in the urine.

LIVER FUNCTION TESTS

Liver function tests can be divided into four groups:

1. Tests for hepatocellular damage

2. Tests for biliary obstruction

3. Tests for protein synthesis

4. Tests for detoxification

1. Tests for Hepatocellular Damage

- Aspartate transaminase (AST)
- Alanine aminotransferase (ALT)

These enzymes are present in liver cells, and after injury to the cell they are released into circulation. They are excellent and sensitive indicators of damage. Enzyme levels are correlative with the amount of damage to the cell. Elevation of both ALT and AST can occur simultaneously and should be read together; however, ALT is more specific for liver damage.

There may be a higher elevation of AST in alcoholic liver disease. In viral hepatitis these enzymes may be elevated to levels of >20 times the normal level.

- Normal AST: 0–40 IU/L
- Normal ALT: 0–40 IU/L

Etiology of elevation:

- Viral hepatitis
- Alcoholic hepatitis
- Drug-induced hepatitis
- Fatty liver
- Auto-immune hepatitis

2. Tests for Biliary Obstruction

- Bilirubin
- Alkaline phosphatase
- Gamma-glutamyltransferase (GGT)

BILIRUBIN

Total bilirubin

Normal: 0.0–1.2 mg/dL

Etiology of elevation:

- Hepatocellular disease (e.g., hepatitis, cirrhosis)
- Biliary tract obstruction
- Hemolytic

Unconjugated bilirubin

Normal: 0.2–0.8 mg/dL

Etiology of elevation:

- Increased production (e.g., hemolysis)
- Impaired hepatic uptake
- Decreased conjugation

Conjugated bilirubin

Normal: 0.1–0.2 mg/dL

Etiology of elevation:

- Intrahepatic cholestasis—a defect in the excretion of bilirubin from the liver cells from:
  - Hepatocellular disease
  - Hepatitis
  - Drug-induced cholestasis
  - Primary biliary cirrhosis
- Extra hepatic cause of obstruction:
  - Gallstones
  - Pancreatic cancer
  - Tumors of the bile duct

ALKALINE PHOSPHATASE

Normal: 25–100 IU/L   (20 - 90)

Alkaline phosphatase is elevated in obstructive liver disease. However, as alkaline phosphatase comes from both bone and the placenta, one has to be certain of the source. If all other liver tests are abnormal, the most likely source is liver. However, if there is an isolated increase of alkaline phosphatase while all other liver enzymes/tests are normal, it is probably a bone abnormality. At this point, a GGT analysis should be performed.

If the GGT is elevated, the alkaline phosphatase is coming from the liver; on the other hand, if the GGT is not elevated, the alkaline phosphatase is coming from the bone. A high level of liver alkaline phosphatase is suggestive of a biliary outflow obstruction. Alkaline phosphatase is elevated in:

- Drug-induced cholestasis
- Primary biliary cirrhosis
- Gallstones
- Pancreatic cancer •
- Tumors of the bile duct
- Sclerosing cholangitis

Bone marrow disease
Paget's
CA

GAMMA-GLUTAMYLTRANSFERASE (GGT)

Normal: 5–45 IU/L

3. Tests for Protein Synthesis

- Prothrombin time
- Albumin

PROTHROMBIN TIME

Normal: 11–13 seconds

Although this is a well-known test of coagulation, it remains an excellent liver function test because many of the coagulation factors are manufactured in the liver. Therefore, a prolonged prothrombin time is very suggestive of liver dysfunction. A simultaneous vitamin K deficiency must be excluded.

ALBUMIN

Normal: 3.5–5.5 g/dL

Albumin is made in the liver and is a major contributor to oncotic pressure, which is essential for normal blood circulation; a decreased level denotes liver impairment. Due to the liver's vast reserve, albumin levels do not decrease until late in the disease. Hypoalbuminemia must be ruled out as a result of loss secondary to kidney dysfunction, from exudation of damaged tissue or from malnutrition.
Etiology of decreased levels:

- Liver cell dysfunction

- Renal loss, as in nephrotic syndrome

- Malnutrition

- Exudation from damaged tissue (e.g., crush injury, burns)

4. Tests for Detoxification

- Serum ammonia

SERUM AMMONIA

One of the most vital protective functions of the liver is the conversion of ammonia to a relatively harmless compound called urea. In advanced liver failure, ammonia will increase and BUN will decrease. This is usually accompanied by signs of hepatic encephalopathy and is typically a terminal event.

ADDITIONAL ISSUES IN THE DIAGNOSIS OF LIVER DISEASE BY LABORATORY TESTING

Additional issues in the diagnosis of liver disease by laboratory testing include the following:

Viral Hepatitis

When viral hepatitis is suspected, liver tests will show marked (up to 20 times) elevation of ALT and AST with a less marked increase of the other liver test values. A viral hepatitis panel should be ordered for proper diagnosis.

Alcoholic Hepatitis

Both AST and ALT are moderately increased but AST is more increased and GGT elevation is correlative with the length and severity of the ETOH (alcohol) abuse.

Jaundice

If there is an increase in the total bilirubin, first assess whether the direct or the indirect bilirubin is increased.

- If the increase is mainly of indirect bilirubin, hemolysis is the most likely possibility. This should be confirmed by reticulocyte count and haptoglobulin levels.

- If the increase is mainly of direct bilirubin, assess the alkaline phosphatase. Increased alkaline phosphatase suggests an obstruction in the biliary tract. The patient will have whitish (clay-colored) stools and will complain of severe generalized pruritus. In this case, the AST and the ALT are not markedly elevated.

- In hepatocellular jaundice, AST and ALT are increased. Due to edema of the liver cell, there is some obstruction of the intra-cellular bile canaliculated, which results in a minor increase of alkaline phosphatase. In this situation, the prothrombin time is easily increased; if this is a chronic process, the albumin will be decreased.

ILLUSTRATIVE CASE FOR PRACTICE

A 32-year-old male came in with the chief complaints of malaise, loss of appetite, loss of desire to smoke, and vague abdominal discomfort. He was also worried that his eyes appeared more yellow than usual. He had been on vacation in South America for the last three months. There is no significant past history or family history. On PE, the only abnormality noticed is mild jaundice and a slight right upper quadrant tenderness.

Question 1 After the history and physical examination, which of the following laboratory tests would you order?

A. Magnetic resonance imaging (MRI) of the liver.

B. Biopsy of the liver.

C. Chemistry profile.

D. CBC.

The correct response is C.

The history and physical examination are very suggestive of a liver disease as the chemistry profile includes numerous liver tests that would be the correct choice.

The results of the chemistry profile were as follows:

Creatinine, serum	0.64 mg/dL	0.57–1.00
GFR	>59 mL/min	1.73>59
BUN/creatinine ratio	22 mg/dL	8–27
Sodium, serum	141 mmol/L	135–144
Potassium, serum	4.2 mmol/L	3.5–5.2
Chloride, serum	104 mmol/L	96–108
Carbon dioxide, total	24 mmol/L	20–32
Calcium, serum	9.2 mg/dL	8.6–10.2
Phosphorus, serum	3.5 mg/dL	2.5–4.5
Protein, total, serum	6.3 g/dL	6.0–8.5
Albumin, serum	2.9 g/dL	3.5–5.5
Globulin, total	2.4 g/dL	1.5–4.5
A/G ratio	1.6	1.1–2.5
Bilirubin, total	5.6 mg/dL	0.0–1.2
Alkaline phosphatase, serum	100 IU/L	25–100
LDH	200 IU/L	100–250
AST (SGOT)	5600 IU/L (high)	0–40
ALT (SGPT)	7835 IU/L (high)	0–40
Iron, serum	84 ug/dL	35–155

Abbreviations: ALT, alanine aminotransferase (formerly SGPT); AST, aspartate transaminase (formerly SGOT); BUN: blood urea nitrogen; GFR, glomerular filtration rate; LDH: lactate dehydrogenase

Question 1 After reviewing the chemistry profile, what is your conclusion?

A. Viral hepatitis.

B. Hepato-cellular jaundice.

C. There is no evidence of obstructive jaundice.

D. All of the above.

The correct response is A.

While travelling in South America, he may have acquired a form of viral hepatitis, as shown by his high AST/ALT levels.

Question 2 What kind of viral hepatitis does he have?

A. Hepatitis A.

B. Hepatitis B.

C. Hepatitis D.

D. Not enough information to make a diagnosis.

The correct response is D.

Question 3 What test should be ordered next to come up with an answer to question 2?

A. Magnetic resonance imaging (MRI) of the liver.

B. Biopsy of the liver.

C. Hepatitis profile.

D. None of the above.

The correct response is C.

The test comes back in 4 days and the results show that the diagnosis is hepatitis A.

Question 4 How is hepatitis A transmitted?

A. Fecal oral route.

B. Sexually transmitted.

C. By needle sharing.

D. Mosquito bite.

The correct response is A.

Question 5 What is the prognosis of hepatitis A?

A. Good.

B. Very bad.

C. Goes into a chronic danger field.

D. Depends on other concurrent liver disease.

The correct response is A.

TCM PERSPECTIVE

As TCM practitioners we focus heavily upon liver patterns in our diagnosis. In my experience, when we discuss those patterns, the patient can become confused as to what we mean. Are we speaking about the actual organ as it relates to its anatomical structure and function or is it an energetic quality we reference? In my opinion, it is sometimes both. By utilizing laboratory testing a practitioner can observe when a TCM diagnosis and a conventional laboratory value both indicate a liver dysfunction. I have had excellent experience in reducing liver enzymes secondary to various etiologies, using nutrition, herbal remedies and acupuncture as part of the treatment plan. By requesting laboratory studies you are taking an initial step toward providing an integrated approach within your TCM practice. By gaining a more complete understanding of conventional laboratory testing, we can provide evidence for the course of treatment we prescribe and eventually its efficacy.

7

LIPIDS

Evaluation and management of lipid levels are very important in the care of hyperlipidemic patients. Elevated cholesterol, especially of the low density lipoprotein fraction, is a major risk factor for atherosclerotic diseases such as myocardial infarction, stroke, or peripheral vascular disease. Lipid research in the last 50 years has clearly shown the relationship between disease, especially atherosclerosis, and specific fractions of lipids. In this handbook, we will discuss four important lipid fractions:

1. Total cholesterol

2. Low density lipoprotein (LDL)

3. High density lipoprotein (HDL)

4. Triglycerides

The most important and clinically significant correlation of an elevated lipid level is atherosclerosis and thus to atherosclerotic heart diseases (ASHD), namely myocardial infarction, strokes, and peripheral vascular disease. The source of the lipid present in the body is both endogenous and exogenous and is affected both by heredity and lifestyle, mainly diet. To determine lipid levels, all blood testing should be done following an eight-hour fast; however, a longer fast of 14 hours may give even more accurate results. Abstaining from alcohol for at least 24 hours before blood drawing is highly recommended. It is important to remember that other than stress there are five other risk factors commonly associated with atherosclerosis:

1. Family history

2. Hyperlipidemia

3. Smoking

4. Hypertension

5. Uncontrolled diabetes mellitus

In past practice it was common to use ratios of different lipid fractions to determine the degree of risk for developing ASHD. It is now known that the actual numbers are more helpful than the ratios. This book will focus on the specific numbers rather than the ratios.

1. TOTAL CHOLESTEROL
Elevated cholesterol is definitely a risk factor for atherosclerosis and should be lowered to desirable levels with lifestyle changes and medications if necessary.

Desirable level: 140–199 mg/dL

Borderline level: 200–239 mg/dL

High level: >250 mg/dL

Etiology of elevated cholesterol:

- Liver disease, especially biliary cirrhosis
- Nephrotic syndrome
- Chronic renal failure
- Hypothyroidism
- Uncontrolled diabetes mellitus
- Alcoholism
- Pregnancy

Etiology of decreased cholesterol:

- Hyperthyroidism
- Malnutrition and malabsorption
- Megaloblastic anemia
- Chronic obstructive pulmonary disease (COPD)
- Myeloproliferative diseases
- Exogenous estrogen intake

2. LOW DENSITY LIPOPROTEIN (LDL)

A large amount of the circulating cholesterol is present in the LDL fraction. This is the lipid fraction that is most associated with atherosclerosis and has often been called "the bad cholesterol." If two or more risk factors of atherosclerosis exist, the LDL level should be maintained at <100 mg/dL. If coronary artery disease is part of the patient profile, the level should be maintained as close to 70 mg/dL as possible.

Desirable level: <130 mg/dL

Borderline risk: 140–150 mg/dL

High risk: >160 mg/dL

Etiology of elevated LDL:

- Hypothyroidism
- Nephrotic syndrome
- COPD
- Uncontrolled diabetes mellitus
- Multiple myeloma

3. HIGH DENSITY LIPOPROTEIN (HDL)

HDL is a class of lipoprotein that helps the cholesterol transport from peripheral tissue to the liver. In doing so it reduces LDL and thus reduces the risk of atherosclerosis, which is why HDL is often called the "good cholesterol."

Decreased levels of HDL are associated with an increased risk of atherosclerotic diseases, and for the most part appear to be genetically determined.

Normal

Men: 35–65 mg/dL

Women: 35–80 mg/dL

Levels <25 mg/dL increase the risk of ASHD.
Etiology of decreased HDL:

- Tangier disease
- Hyperthyroidism
- Severe liver disease

4. TRIGLYCERIDES

Triglycerides have a lesser role as a causative factor for atherosclerosis versus LDL. Very high levels, >500 mg/dL, may lead to acute pancreatitis. There is a definite correlation between triglyceride level and body weight, and therefore great importance in maintaining appropriate weight.

Desirable level: <150 mg/dL

Borderline level: 150–200 mg/dL

High level: 200 –500 mg/dL

Etiology of elevated levels:

- Liver disease

- Alcoholism

- Uncontrolled diabetes mellitus

- Nephrotic syndrome

- Hypothyroidism

Etiology of decreased levels:

- Malnutrition

- Low fat diet

- Malabsorption

- Hyperthyroidism

TCM PERSPECTIVE

Many patients will present in your TCM practice with metabolic disorders including hyperlipidemia. If you are practicing in a state where you have the right to request laboratory testing, all patients should have, at a minimum, blood tests that include a full lipid profile. If you are not practicing with the right to order, then best practice would be to request a copy of the most recent test from the PCP or specialist. Again, this is a concrete baseline that can be used to justify treatment with acupuncture, herbs, nutrition, and other supplements. In this way, you will be building evidence that Oriental medicine is effective in the treatment of hyperlipidemia, metabolic syndrome, and many other metabolic disorders.

8

ENDOCRINOLOGY

The endocrine system uses hormones that are secreted by the endocrine glands and transported by the circulatory system to target sites. These hormones have a profound influence on the functioning of the body.

This chapter is divided into two sections—the basic science of endocrinology and laboratory tests in the diagnosis of common endocrine diseases.

The secretions of the glands listed below will not be described in detail because diseases pertaining to the endocrine function of these glands are not often seen in a TCM practice setting:

- Pineal

- Thymus

- Kidney

- Heart
- The GI System

BASIC SCIENCE

We will mainly focus on the secretions of the following five glands:

1. Pituitary
2. Thyroid
3. Parathyroid
4. Adrenal
5. Gonads

1. Pituitary

The pituitary is divided into two parts, anterior and posterior. Although the hypothalamus controls many glands, the pituitary is considered a master gland, exerting its control as follows:

SECRETIONS OF THE ANTERIOR PITUITARY

- Adrenocorticotrophic hormone (ACTH) is a trophic hormone of the adrenal gland and controls many of the secretions of the adrenal cortex.

- Thyroid stimulating hormone (TSH) is a trophic hormone of the thyroid gland and controls thyroid secretion.

- Prolactin is a hormone that assists in breast development of the pregnant woman and, ultimately, lactation.

- Growth hormone assists with development and achievement of adult height. It also helps with the metabolism of carbohydrates, fats, and protein.

- Luteinizing hormone (LH) and follicle stimulating hormone (FSH) assist with development of the gonads and their secretions, which are vital for proper reproduction.

SECRETIONS OF THE POSTERIOR PITUITARY

- Anti-diuretic hormone (ADH) works on the distal part of the nephron, and controls fluid balance by adjusting the amount excreted in the urine. The absence of ADH results in diabetes insipidus.

- Oxytocin causes the contraction of the uterus during labor and assists in the eventual birth.

2. Thyroid

The thyroid gland controls multiple metabolic functions of the body by secreting thyroxine (T4) and triiodothyronine (T3). These functions include: heat production, mentation, bodyweight maintenance, energy supply, and fatigue prevention. There is a third hormone secretion by the thyroid gland called calcitonin. This functions to lower calcium when it is elevated. Unfortunately, in pathological conditions where the parathyroid hormone causes hypercalcemia, calcitonin is incapable of correcting the problem.

3. Parathyroid

The parathyroid gland produces parathyroid hormone (PTH), and, along with vitamin D, maintains the optimum level of calcium in the human body. Whenever calcium levels fall, PTH is secreted. This stimulates the osteoclast cells in the bone, causing a microscopic breakdown of the bone and the release of calcium, thus adjusting the level.

4. Adrenal

The adrenal gland is divided into the cortex and the medulla. The medulla's function is focused upon control of all autonomic functions. The main hormones produced are epinephrine and norepinephrine. The three layers of the cortex are:

1. Zona Glomerulosa—produces aldosterone and functions to reabsorb sodium at the nephron. This exchange of sodium for potassium functions to maintain sodium levels and adequate fluid volume.

2. Zona Fasciculata—produces cortisol, a very important hormone with a function to protect the body from stress.

3. Zona Reticularis—produces androgenic sex hormone, which in females is the main androgenic hormone.

5. Gonads

THE TESTES

The leydig cells of the testicle produce testosterone under the stimulus of pituitary LH. Seminiferous tubular cells produce sperm under the stimulus of pituitary FSH.

THE OVARY

The primordial follicle cells under the stimulus of pituitary FSH produce estrogen, especially in the proliferative phase of the menstrual cycle. Following ovulation, which is caused by the pituitary LH surge, the primordial follicle becomes the corpus luteum and begins secreting progesterone in addition to estrogen.

LABORATORY TESTS IN THE DIAGNOSIS OF COMMON ENDOCRINE DISEASES
Diseases of the Thyroid Gland

- Primary hyperthyroidism
  - Graves' disease
- Primary hypothyroidism
  - Hashimoto's disease
- Goiter

THYROID LEVELS

The thyroid gland secretes two thyroid hormones: thyroxine (T4) and triiodothyronine (T3). T4 is a less active hormone and acts as a precursor of T3. Both hormones are carried in the blood in two forms. The protein-bound form acts as a reserve and the free form is the active hormone.

In the past, laboratory assessment could only measure total T4, which is the summation of the protein-bound and free form. This value was often misleading. Nowadays, laboratory assessment is capable of measuring free thyroxine (Free T4). This form is the most accurate representation of the thyroid status and is the only form that should be used to assess the state of the thyroid.

The thyroid gland secretes thyroxine in response to TSH, which is secreted by the anterior pituitary gland. A general guideline in determining thyroid levels is as follows: If TSH is elevated, the initial interpretation is that of hypothyroidism as the pituitary is identifying through its information feedback loop that there is too little thyroxine and is requesting additional thyroxine be secreted. Likewise, if the TSH is low, then the initial interpretation is hyperthyroidism or excess exogenous hormone replacement, as the pituitary is identifying too much thyroxine in the blood.

The thyroid gland secretion, T4, which is ultimately inactive or what is known as "protein bound," must be converted into T3, which could be said is "free or unbound." This biologically active T3 stimulates the metabolism of multiple tissues in the body and is what could be functionally low, causing symptoms that would otherwise not be identified with testing TSH or total T4/T3. Due to the ability to test both total and free thyroid hormones, it is important to remember that when we suspect hyperthyroidism or hypothyroidism, we measure the free hormone levels and not the total levels. The TSH as an individual test is excellent; however, the underlying picture will not become apparent until you assess the free levels.

PRIMARY HYPERTHYROIDISM (E.G., GRAVES' DISEASE)

Usual tests ordered: Free T4 and TSH

Free T4

Normal: 0.82–1.77 ug/dL

TSH

Normal: 0.450–4.500 uIU/mL

If Free T4 is elevated and TSH is decreased, the diagnosis is probably primary hyperthyroidism.

About 10% of patients with hyperthyroidism have T3 toxicosis. If a patient appears clinically to show hyperthyroidism but the Free T4 is not increased, a free triiodothyronine (Free T3) test should be ordered. If the person has this rarer variant called T3 toxicosis, the Free T3 will be increased and TSH will be suppressed.

PRIMARY HYPOTHYROIDISM

Usual tests ordered: Free T4 and TSH

If Free T4 is decreased and TSH is elevated, the diagnosis is most likely primary hypothyroidism.

Hashimoto's Disease

This is the most common form of auto-immune thyroiditis that leads to hypothyroidism. In many hypothyroid patients, thyroid antibodies are checked to find the etiology of the hypothyroid state. Diagnosing Hashimoto's disease includes testing for those antibodies, and if they are elevated, then the hypothyroidism would be positive for Hashimoto's disease.

Monitoring Hormone Levels of a Hypothyroid Patient

Usual tests ordered: Free T4 and TSH

Most patients will be medically managed by their PCP or endocrinologist. The laboratory tests to order are, again, Free T4 and TSH. TSH can be used alone to adjust the exogenous hormone dosage. If the TSH is still high, the replacement dosage needs to be increased. If the TSH is decreased, the replacement dosage needs to be decreased. The Free T4 may provide additional information for finer adjustments.

GOITER

This is a nonspecific term denoting an enlargement of the thyroid. It does not state the functional status of the thyroid, so proper investigation is needed. Common thinking is that goiter is caused by an iodine deficiency; however, iodine replacement is highly controversial and should be medically managed.

Diseases of the Parathyroid Gland

- Hyperparathryroidism
- Hypoparathyroidism

PTH is secreted by the parathyroid gland whenever serum calcium is low. This stimulates the osteoclast cells in the bone to break down microscopic amounts of bone cells and release calcium. For diagnosis of hyperparathyroidism or hypoparathyroidism, both calcium levels and PTH should be tested.

HYPERPARATHYROIDISM

Hyperparathyroidism should be suspected if laboratory results show an elevated calcium level. The common clinical presentation is the presence of kidney stones and/or bone pathology (i.e., osteoporosis, often accompanied by low phosphates).

Usual tests ordered: PTH and serum calcium

PTH

Normal: 10.0–55.0 pg/mL

Serum calcium

· Normal: 8.7–10.2 mg/dL

If the serum calcium level and PTH level are increased, the diagnosis is most likely hyperparathyroidism.

Note: Isolated elevation of PTH should never be used to make a diagnosis of hyperparathyroidism.

HYPOPARATHYROIDISM

Usual tests ordered: PTH and serum calcium

If the serum calcium level and PTH level are decreased, the diagnosis is most likely hypoparathyroidism. Commonly there is a past history of neck surgery.

Diseases of the Adrenal Gland

- Cushing's syndrome
- Addison's disease

CUSHING'S SYNDROME

Elevated cortisol is the primary sign.

Etiology of elevated levels:

- Excess adrenal production of cortisol
- Excess ACTH production by the anterior pituitary
- Excessive exogenous intake of cortisone such as medication
- Production of excess ACTH by a tumor (paraneoplastic syndrome)

Diagnosis should be divided into two parts.

1. Establish the presence of Cushing's syndrome by measuring urinary free cortisol.

2. Identify the etiology of excess cortisol, possibly found in the history.

    Usual tests ordered: ACTH

    ACTH

    Normal: 10.0–60.0 pg/mL

Elevated ACTH suggests a pituitary or paraneoplastic issue, whereas decreased ACTH suggests an adrenal pathology.

ADDISON'S DISEASE

Addison's disease is characterized by hypofunction of adrenal cortex.

Usual tests ordered: ACTH and serum cortisol

ACTH

Normal: 10.0–60.0 pg/mL

Serum cortisol

Normal: 5–25 mcg/dL (am); 2–14 mcg/dL (pm)

Serum cortisol is decreased, whereas serum ACTH is elevated; therefore the diagnosis is most likely Addison's disease.

Diseases of the Pituitary Gland

- Panhypopituitarism
- Pituitary tumors

PANHYPOPITUITARISM (E.G., SHEEHAN'S SYNDROME)

Usual tests ordered: Free T4 and TSH

Though all the pituitary hormones could be assessed, typically only one or two pituitary hormones and the hormones of the trophic gland are tested. For example, if a Free T4 is checked and is decreased with TSH being simultaneously decreased, it would suggest that the pituitary is malfunctioning.

PITUITARY TUMORS

These are often suspected when a patient presents with headaches, hemianopsia, and pituitary hormone abnormality, usually involving one hormone that is being secreted excessively.

Diseases of the Gonads

Normal hormone levels are as follows:

LH

Female menstruating:

Follicular phase: 2.0–15.0 mIU/mL

Ovulatory phase: 22.0–105.0 mIU/mL

Luteal phase: 0.6–19.0 mIU/mL

Postmenopausal: 16.0–64.0 mIU/mL

Male: 2.0–12.0 mIU/mL

FSH

Female menstruating:

Follicular phase: 3.0–20.0 mIU/mL

Ovulatory phase: 29.0–26.0 mIU/mL

Luteal phase: 1.0–12.0 mIU/mL

Postmenopausal: 18.0–153.0 mIU/mL

Male: 1.0–12.0 mIU/mL

In males:

Sperm count

Normal: >15 million/mL

TESTICULAR FAILURE

Usual tests ordered include: serum testosterone, luteinizing hormone, follicle stimulating hormone and sperm count

In primary testicular failure, testosterone will be decreased, and LH will be elevated.

MENOPAUSE

In menopause FSH is increased, LH is elevated, and estrogen is decreased.

Usual test ordered: FSH

FSH

Female menstruating:

Follicular phase: 3.0–20.0 mIU/mL

Ovulatory phase: 29.0–26.0 mIU/mL

Luteal phase: 1.0–12.0 mIU/mL

Postmenopausal: 18.0–153.0 mIU/mL

Male: 1.0–12.0 mIU/mL

ILLUSTRATIVE CASE FOR PRACTICE

This 42-year-old female came in with complaints of tiredness, feeling cold, dry skin, constipation, and heavy menstrual periods.

PH: Gravida 1; parity 1. Patient was hospitalized five years ago for a month because of depression; however, she does not feel that is a problem at present.

FH: Both mother and grandmother had history of goiter. Her grandmother had surgery to remove her goiter.

SH: The patient smokes cigarettes—one pack of 20 per day—and works as a secretary. She is married and lives with her husband and child.

PE: Other than some conjunctival pallor and a large diffuse goiter three times normal size, the patient's physical examination is normal.

Question 1 Based on the history and physical examination, which test would you order initially?

A. Total T3, T4.

B. Free T4 and TSH.

C. Refer the patient for depression.

D. Chemistry profile.

The correct response is B.

The history and physical examination are strongly suggestive of familial thyroid pathology, and her symptoms, including the presence of a goiter, suggest a hypothyroid state. Total T3 and T4 is an outdated test and should be replaced by Free T4 and TSH.

Results of the above tests are:

Free T4: 2.8 ug/dL (low)

TSH: 33 uIU/mL (high)

Question 2 What is your conclusion from the blood tests?

A. Hypothyroidism.

B. Hyperthyroidism.

C. Normothyroidism.

D. Pituitary disorder.

The correct response is A

Low Free T4 with a high TSH is very suggestive of primary hypothyroidism.

The result was discussed with the patient. She wanted to know why she, her mother, and grandmother all have thyroid pathologies and if there is any way to test for it.

Question 3 What are your thoughts?

A. She has Hashimoto's thyroiditis.

B. Her mother and grandmother also had Hashimoto's thyroiditis.

C. Blood test for Hashimoto's thyroiditi, to include microsomal thyroid antibodies, is indicated.

D. All of the above.

The correct response is D.

Patient was referred out to an internist, who started her on Synthroid 25 mcg/qd. She returned for a follow-up five weeks later, feeling much better.

Question 4 To assess how she is doing and to adjust the dose of her Synthroid, which test should be ordered?

A. T3 and T4.

B. T4.

C. Free T4 and TSH.

D. Chemistry profile.

The correct response is C.

If the TSH level remains elevated, the patient needs more Synthroid. If the TSH level is too low, the dose of Synthroid needs to be reduced.

The test results are:

Free T4: decreased

TSH: elevated

Thyroid microsomal antibodies: very high level

Question 5 What is your conclusion from the test results?

A. Hypothyroidism secondary to Hashimoto's thyroiditis.

B. The patient has depression.

C. Hashimoto's disease should be treated with immuno-suppressive medications.

The correct response is A.

Her dose of exogenous hormone replacement was adjusted and the patient returned in six weeks, stating that she was feeling even better. This auto-immune type of thyroiditis can be strongly hereditary and would explain the familial tendency.

TCM PERSPECTIVE

Management of hormone-based complaints is common in a TCM practice but can be very tricky to balance between the PCP, endocrinologist and the TCM practitioner. By understanding the various biochemical mechanisms underlying these complaints, you can better stand your ground when prescribing an herbal, glandular, or nutritional supplement for your patient. Oriental medicine effectively treats these conditions and it is time that we as practitioners begin to document our successes so that we can share the information with the public. Having a scientific background will assist you in feeling confident and proving your point to the community at large.

PRACTICE QUESTIONS

Q1 A WBC count of 100,000 is suggestive of:

A. Infection.

B. Leukemia.

C. Normalcy.

D. Dehydration.

Q2 The best way to check for hemolysis is to:

A. Check for blood in stool.

B. Check for blood in urine.

C. Do a reticulocyte count.

D. Measure LDL.

Q3 The MCV that suggests vitamin B12 deficiency anemia is:

A. 12.

B. 14.

C. 62.

D. 110.

Q4 The MCV value that suggests microcytic anemia is:

A. 12.

B. 14.

C. 62.

D. 110.

Q5 In anemia of bone marrow failure:

A. Reticulocyte count is decreased.

B. Hypersegmented polymorphs are present.

C. TIBC is increased.

D. Iron is decreased.

Q6 An increase in reticulocyte count is seen in:

A. Hemolytic anemia.

B. Obstructive jaundice.

C. Cancer of the head of the pancreas.

D. All of the above.

Q7 Which organ helps remove senescent RBCs?

A. Liver.

B. Kidney.

C. Spleen.

D. Thymus.

Q8 An increase in eosinophil count suggests:

A. Allergy.

B. Infection.

C. Cancer.

D. None of the above.

Q9 The precursor cell for the platelet is called:

A. Proerythroblast.

B. Megakaryocyte.

C. Reticulocyte.

D. B cell.

Q10 Causes of hemolysis include:

A. Mismatched blood transfusion.

B. Sickle cell disease.

C. Thalassemia.

D. All of the above.

Q11 On dipstick urine analysis, the presence of nitrites suggests:

A. Cancer.

B. Kidney stones.

C. Infection.

D. Kidney failure.

Q12 Types of kidney stones include:

A. Calcium carbonate.

B. Uric acid.

C. Triple phosphate.

D. All of the above.

Q13 The kidney excretes nitrogenous wastes in the form of BUN. This is made in the:

A. Liver.

B. Kidney.

C. Heart.

D. Colon.

Q14 Other than renal failure, an increase of BUN can also be seen in:

A. Acute myocardial infarction.

B. GI bleed.

C. Liver disease.

D. Hyperthyroidism.

Q15 Etiologies of hematuria include:

A. Torsion of the testicle.

B. Kidney stone.

C. Diabetes mellitus.

D. Chronic renal failure.

Q16 Creatinine clearance is a good test to assess:

A. Renal threshold.

B. Filtration capacity.

C. Glomerular filtration rate.

D. Renal blood flow.

Q17 How much urine does the kidney create in 24 hours?

A. 80 L.

B. 1.5 L.

C. 5 L.

D. 25 L.

Q18 In renal failure, serum potassium level is:

A. Decreased.

B. Increased.

C. Does not change.

D. Depends on the level of magnesium.

Q19 If urine glucose is detected on dipstick analysis, it means that:

A. The patient may be pre-diabetic, and serum glucose levels should be assessed.

B. The patient is diabetic.

C. The patient has a UTI.

D. The patient has nephrotic syndrome.

Q20 In renal failure, the cause of anemia is:

A. Bleeding.

B. Iron deficiency.

C. Erythropoetin deficiency.

D. Bone marrow suppression.

Q21 Low serum potassium is seen with:

A. Volume depletion.

B. Diuretic use.

C. Congestive heart failure (CHF).

D. Liver disease.

Q22 High levels of serum potassium are seen in:

A. Kidney failure.

B. Increased ingestion of potassium-containing food.

C. Liver failure.

D. Heart failure.

Q23 High serum calcium and the presence of a kidney stone are suggestive of:

A. Volume depletion.

B. Hyperparathyroidism.

C. Renal failure.

D. Cancer of the head of the pancreas.

Q24 Etiology of low magnesium includes:

A. Malabsorption syndrome.

B. Renal failure.

C. CHF.

D. Hepatoma.

Q25 Which of the following is true in severe volume depletion?

A. Serum sodium may be increased.

B. Angiotensin 2 is increased.

C. Anti-diuretic hormone is increased.

D. All of the above.

Q26 Normal pH of human blood is:

A. 7.35.

B. 2.

C. 9.

D. Acidotic.

Q27 High Hb1AC is suggestive of:

A. Good diabetic control.

B. Poor diabetic control.

C. Early kidney failure.

D. Diabetes and anemia.

Q28 To detect early diabetic nephropathy, which one of the following should be checked?

A. Serum BUN.

B. Serum potassium.

C. Urine microalbumin.

D. Serum creatinine.

Q29 To make a diagnosis of diabetes mellitus:

A. Check urinary glucose.

B. Check HbA1c.

C. Check fasting blood glucose.

D. Perform a glucose tolerance test.

Q30 The most common cause of hypoglycemia is:

A. Treatment of diabetes mellitus.

B. Starvation.

C. Alcohol intoxication.

D. Acute pancreatitis.

Q31 Ketonuria is seen in:

A. Renal failure.

B. Starvation.

C. A result of protein breakdown.

D. UTI.

Q32 GAD and islet cell antibody tests are performed to:

A. Make a diagnosis of diabetes mellitus.

B. Evaluate the degree of diabetic control.

C. Determine whether the patient has type 1 or type 2 diabetes mellitus.

D. Check for complications of diabetes mellitus.

Q33 Which one of the following is not a chronic complication of diabetes mellitus?

A. Kidney failure.

B. Liver failure.

C. Blindness.

D. Amputation of the lower extremities.

Q34 In type 1 diabetes mellitus:

A. There is an excess of insulin.

B. No insulin is secreted.

C. Insulin receptors are non-functional.

D. There is severe insulin resistance.

Q35 A 45-year-old female has obstruction of her bile duct with a gallstone resulting in severe jaundice. She will also have an increase in:

A. AST.

B. Alkalinephosphatase.

C. Albumin.

D. BUN.

Q36 Bilirubin is formed from:

A. Nucleus of the cell.

B. RBC.

C. Bacteria.

D. Amino acids.

Q37 Elevated alkaline phosphatase levels can be seen in:

A. Bone disease.

B. Kidney disease.

C. Liver disease.

D. Bone disease and kidney disease.

Q38 In severe liver failure:

A. BUN is increased.

B. Ammonia is increased.

C. Bilirubin is decreased.

D. Glucose is increased.

Q39 In viral hepatitis, there is a marked increase in:

A. Alkaline phosphatase.

B. AST and ALT.

C. Reticulocyte count.

D. Albumin.

Q40 Cancer of the head of the pancreas will often present with increase in:

A. AST.

B. Alkaline phosphatase.

C. Albumin.

D. BUN.

Q41 What is the most likely diagnosis in a 40-year-old woman with the following laboratory results?

Sodium	140 mmol/L
Potassium	4 mmol/L
Calcium	8 mg/mL
Bun	24 mg/dL
Creatinine	2 mg/dL
AST	44 IU/L
ALT	34 IU/L

Total bilirubin   12 mg/dL (high)

Direct bilirubin   11 mg/dL (high)

Indirect bilirubin   1 mg/dL

A. Viral hepatitis.

B. Alcoholic hepatitis.

C. Obstruction due to gallstones.

D. Mono hepatitis.

Q42 The most damaging fraction of cholesterol is:

A. HDL.

B. LDL.

C. Very low density lipoprotein (VLDL).

D. Chylomicron.

Q43 Before blood is drawn to analyze for lipid levels, the patient should fast for:

A. 12 hours.

B. 6 hours.

C. 8 hours.

D. No fasting is necessary.

Q44 High levels of cholesterol are seen with:

A. Hyperthyroidism.

B. Hypothyroidism.

C. Hypertension.

D. Addison's disease.

Q45 Very high levels of triglyceride might result in:

A. Cerebrovascular accident.

B. Renal failure.

C. Acute pancreatitis.

D. Hyper viscocity syndrome.

Q46 Prior to having blood drawn for lipid assay, it is advisable to:

A. Abstain from alcohol for 12 hours.

B. Abstain from alcohol for 4 hours.

C. Abstain from sex.

D. Abstain from intense physical activity.

Q47 High serum calcium is seen in people who have:

A. Hyperparathyriodism.

B. Been taking large amounts of calcium.

C. Malabsorption.

D. All of the above.

Q48 Aldosterone causes which one of the following:

A. Potassium retention.

B. Sodium retention.

C. Calcium retention.

D. Magnesium retention.

Q49 The best test for hypothyroidism is:

A. T3.

B. T4.

C. Free T4 and Free T3.

D. Free T4 and TSH.

Q50 The test usually done to make a diagnosis of menopause is:

A. FSH.

B. Pap smear.

C. HDL.

D. Prolactin.

Q51 In primary testicular failure, as in Klinefelter syndrome, the LH level is:

A. Increased.

B. Decreased.

C. Unchanged.

D. Undetectable.

Answer Key

1. A, 2. C, 3. C, 4. D, 5. C,
6. A, 7. A, 8. C, 8. A, 9. B,
10. D, 11. C, 12. D, 13. A,
14. B, 15. B, 16. C, 17. A,
18. B, 19. A, 20. C, 21. B,
22. A, 23. B, 24. A, 25. D
26. A, 27. B, 28. C, 29. C,
30. A, 31. B, 32. C, 33. B,
34. B, 35. B, 36. B, 37. D,
38. B, 39. B, 40. B, 41. C,
42. B, 43. A, 44. B, 45. A,
46. A, 47. A, 48. D, 49. C,
50. A, 51. A

FURTHER READING

Fischbach, F. and Dunning, M.B. (2008) *A Manual of Laboratory and Diagnostic Tests.* Baltimore, MD: Lippincott Williams & Wilkins.

Longo D., Fauci A., Kasper, D., Hauser, S., Jameson J., and Loscalzo, J. (2011) *Harrison's Principles of Internal Medicine,* 18th edn. New York, NY: McGraw-Hill Professional.

Lord, R. and Bralley, J.A. (eds) (2008) *Laboratory Evaluations for Integrative and Functional Medicine Revised,* 2nd edn. Duluth, GA: Metametrix.

Lippincott Williams & Wilkins (2010) *Professional Guide to Signs and Symptoms.* Baltimore, MD: Lippincott Williams & Wilkins.

Porter, R.S. (ed.) (2011) *The Merck Manual.* Whitehouse Station, NJ: Merck Sharp & Dohme Corp.

Venes, D. (ed.) (2013) *Tabers Cyclopedic Medical Dictionary.* Philadelphia, PA: F.A. Davis Company.

GLOSSARY

References: http://medical-dictionary.thefreedictionary.com
http://www.merriam-webster.com/medical

Acute phase reactant A substance in the blood that increases as a response to an acute condition such as infection, injury, tissue destruction, and some cancers.

Addison's disease A disorder involving disrupted functioning of the part of the adrenal gland called the cortex.

Albumin The major plasma protein responsible for transport of large anions.

Alkaline phosphatase An enzyme with an activity in serum that is useful in diagnosing many diseases.

Anal fissure A cleft or groove in the anus.

Anemia Reduction below normal of the number of erythrocytes, quantity of hemoglobin, or volume of packed red cells.

Aplastic Unable to form or regenerate tissue.

Arterial blood gas The oxygen and carbon dioxide content of arterial blood measured to assess the adequacy of oxygenation and the acid base status of the body.

Aspiration The drawing of a foreign substance or removal of a fluid from a body cavity, such as a biopsy.

Atherosclerotic diseases Disease pertaining to atherosclerosis, which is the plaque build-up on the inside of blood vessels.

Auto-immune Directed against the body's own tissues.

Auto-immune disease Any group of disorders in which tissue injury is associated with humoral- or cell-mediated responses to the body's own constituents.

Best practice A technique, method, or process which conventional wisdom regards as more effective at delivering a particular outcome than any other technique, method, or process when applied to a particular condition or circumstance.

Bilirubin The yellow breakdown of normal heme, which is the principal constituent of RBCs. It is responsible for the yellow discoloration in jaundice.

Blood urea nitrogen (BUN) This test is a measure of the amount of nitrogen in the blood in the form of urea.

Calcitonin A hormone produced by the thyroid, which acts to reduce blood calcium in opposition to the parathyroid hormone (PTH).

Cardiac arrhythmia Any condition where there is abnormal electrical activity in the heart.

Chronic obstructive pulmonary disease (COPD) Refers to chronic bronchitis and emphysema, which co-exist in the lungs leading to airway narrowing and constriction, causing shortness of breath (SOB).

Cockcroft–Gault formula Calculation to estimate the glomerular filtration rate (GFR).

Conjunctiva A clear mucus membrane consisting of cells that cover the sclera of the eye and lines the inside of the eyelids.

Conventional medicine The expected norm of Western medical approaches to healing and wellness.

Cortisol Steroid hormone produced by the adrenal gland.

C-Peptide Participates in the biosynthesis of insulin. It is an important link between the A- and B-chains of insulin, and facilitates processing.

Creatinine A breakdown product of creatine phosphate in muscle, it is filtered out of the blood by the kidneys.

Cushing's syndrome A hormone disorder caused by high levels of cortisol in the blood.

Diabetes insipidus Diabetes caused most commonly by a deficiency in arginine vasopressin (AVP), also known as antidiuretic hormone (ADH).

Diabetes mellitus A group of metabolic diseases in which the individual has elevated blood sugar, due to either the lack of insulin production or the lack of response/sensitivity by the cells to insulin.

Diabetic ketoacidosis Potentially life-threatening complication in patients with diabetes mellitus types 1 and 2. It results from a shortage of insulin; in response, the body burns fatty acids for fuel, resulting in increased ketones.

Electrolytes Any of the various ions that are required by cells to regulate the electric charge and flow of water molecules across the cell membrane. Examples include sodium, potassium, and chloride.

Endocrinology The study of glands and hormones of the body and their related disorders.

Endogenous Produced from within an organism, cell, or tissue.

Endoscopy Visual examination of a hollow organ.

Etiology The cause or origin of a disease or disorder as determined by medical diagnosis.

ETOH Abbreviation for ethanol/alcohol (drinking alcohol).

Evidence Data that are for the purpose of supporting or rejecting a hypothesis, typically through observation or created experiments.

Exogenous Coming from the outside. For example, medication delivered orally, by injection, or intravenously is considered exogenous.

Gestational diabetes mellitus A condition in which women without previously diagnosed diabetes exhibit high blood glucose levels during pregnancy.

Glomerular filtration rate (GFR) A measure of kidney functioning, it is a test used to determine renal function status.

Glucagon A hormone secreted by the pancreas that raises blood sugar levels.

Glucose-6-phosphate dehydrogenase deficiency (G6PD) The most common human enzyme defect, it is involved in the pentose phosphate pathway.

Glutamic acid decarboxylase (GAD) An enzyme catalyst.

Glycosuria The excretion of glucose into the urine.

Goiter A swelling in the thyroid gland.

Gravida The number of times a woman has been pregnant.

Growth hormone (GH) A protein-based peptide hormone that stimulates growth, cell reproduction, and regeneration in humans and other animals.

Haptoglobin A normal plasma protein that functions to bind hemoglobin in the bloodstream.

Hashimoto's thyroiditis Inflammation of thyroid gland and destruction of cells from an auto-immune disorder.

Hematocrit Measurement of how much space in the blood is occupied by RBCs.

Hemianopsia Loss of vision in one half of the visual field of one or both eyes.

Hemoccult Trademark for a guaiac reagent strip test for occult blood.

Hemochromatosis An inherited blood disorder that causes the body to retain excessive amounts of iron.

Hemoglobin The oxygen-carrying pigment of erythrocytes.

Hemoglobin A1C Glycosylated hemoglobin, which is helpful in evaluating effective control of diabetes.

Hemolytic anemia A disorder in which RBCs are destroyed prematurely.

Hemorrhoid Prolapse of the anal cushion, resulting in bleeding and swelling.

Hepatic encephalopathy Degenerative brain disease occurring secondary to advanced liver disease.

Hepatitis Inflammation of the liver.

Hormone replacement therapy Use of synthetic or natural hormones to make up for the lack of hormones made in the body.

Hyperaldosteronism A disorder that is defined by the overproduction of aldosterone.

Hypercalcemia Abnormally high level of calcium in the blood.

Hyperkalemia Abnormally high level of potassium in the blood.

Hyperlipidemia Elevated concentrations of any or all lipids in the plasma.

Hypermagnesemia Abnormally large magnesium content of the blood plasma.

Hypernatremia Abnormal elevation of sodium in the blood plasma.

Hyperperfusion Excess passage of fluid through the vessels of a specific organ.

Hypersplenism Disorder that causes the spleen to rapidly and prematurely destroy blood cells.

Hypervitaminosis D Toxic effect of ingesting large amounts of vitamin D.

Hypoalbuminemia Abnormally low level of albumin in the blood.

Hypocalcemia Abnormally low level of calcium in the blood.

Hypokalemia Abnormally low level of potassium in the blood.

Hypomagnesemia Abnormally low level of magnesium in the blood.

Hyponatremia Abnormally low level of sodium in the blood.

Hypoproteinemia Abnormally low level of total protein in the blood.

Hypovolemia Low volume relating to the human body.

Intramuscular (IM) injection Injection of a substance directly into the muscle.

Intravenous (IV) Administration of substances directly into the vein.

Intrinsic factor Glycoprotein produced by parietal cells of the stomach.

Insulin A hormone that is central to regulating carbohydrate and fat metabolism.

Inulin Naturally occurring polysaccharide produced by plants.

Islet cell auto-antibody Antibody active against a pancreatic islet cell.

Jaundice Yellowish pigmentation of the skin, tissues and some body fluids caused by a disruption in the discharge of bile, indicating liver disease.

Ketone body One of three organic compounds that accumulate in the blood or urine in abnormal amounts in impaired conditions such as diabetes.

Laryngospasm Spasmodic closure of the larynx.

Leucopenia Abnormal number of circulating white blood cells.

Leukemoid reaction A reaction resembling leukemia but not involving the same changes in the blood-forming organs.

Lipids Combined with proteins and carbohydrates compose the principal structure of living cells.

Malignant Tending to produce death or deterioration.

Mean corpuscular volume (MCV) Volume of the average red blood cell.

Metabolic diseases An impairment of the normal state of metabolic functions due to specific pathogens or inherent defects.

Microalbumin Microscopic traces of albumin.

Myeloproliferative A disorder marked by excessive proliferation of bone marrow elements.

Myocardial infarction Heart attack.

Nephron A single excretory unit of the vertebrate kidney.

Nephropathy An abnormal state of the kidney.

Nephrotic syndrome An abnormal condition marked by a deficiency of albumin.

Neuropathy An abnormal and usually degenerative state of the nervous system.

Ophthalmic Of, relating, or situated near the eye.

Orthostatic hypotension Low blood pressure related to an erect posture.

Pancreatitis Inflammation of the pancreas.

Parathyroid hormone (PTH) Hormone of the parathyroid gland that regulates the metabolism of calcium.

Parity Number of live births or number of times a female has given birth, counting multiple births as one and usually including still births.

Peripheral vascular disease Vascular disease such as Raynaud's, affecting blood vessels outside the heart, specifically those vessels supplying the extremities.

Pernicious anemia Severe hyperchromic anemia with decreased intrinsic factor production.

Polycythemia vera A myeloproliferative disease of unknown cause characterized by an increase of total blood volume and viscosity.

Polydipsia Excessive abnormal thirst.

Polyuria Excessive secretion of urine.

Postprandial Occurring after a meal.

Primary care physician Skilled healthcare professional trained and licensed to practice medicine, usually a non-specialist.

Primary disease A disease arising spontaneously and not associated with or caused by previous disease.

Proerythroblast Hemocytoblast that gives rise to erythroblasts.

Purpura Any of several hemorrhagic states characterized by patches of purplish discoloration.

Pyelonephritis Inflammation of both parenchyma of a kidney and the lining of its renal pelvis secondary to bacterial infection.

Quantitative protein Relating to or involving quality or kind changes in proteins.

Reticulocyte An immature red blood cell that appears during regeneration of lost blood.

Reticuloendothelial (RE) system A system of cells of varying lineage that were originally grouped together because of their supposed phagocytic properties.

Retinopathy Any of various non-inflammatory disorders of the retina.

Rheumatology A medical scientific discipline dealing with rheumatic diseases.

Secondary disease A disease that follows and results from an earlier disease.

Serum A clear yellowish fluid that remains in blood plasma after clotting factors have been removed.

Sign Objective evidence of disease, especially as observed and interpreted by the physician.

Sublingual Situated or administered under the tongue.

Symptom Subjective evidence of disease as observed by the patient.

Syncope Loss of consciousness resulting from insufficient blood flow to the brain.

Syndrome of inappropriate ADH (SIADH) Defined by hyponatremia and hypo-osmolality resulting from inappropriate continued secretion or action of the hormone.

Synthroid Prescription drug, also known as levothyroxine, which is used as hormone replacement for deficient thyroid hormone.

Thalassemia Any group of inherited hypochromic anemias, occurring especially in individuals from the Mediterranean.

T3 toxicosis Pathological condition of excess triiodothyronine.

Thrombocytopenia Persistent decrease in the number of blood platelets.

Troponin A protein of muscle that together with tropomyosin forms a regulatory complex controlling the interaction of actin and myosin.

Urinalysis The physical, chemical and microscopic analysis of urine.

Urobilinogen Any of several chromogens that are reduction products of bilirubin.

Vasoconstriction Narrowing of the lumen of blood vessels, especially as a result of vasomotor action.

Very low density lipoprotein (VLDL) A fat transporter that converts in the bloodstream to low density lipoprotein (LDL).

INDEX

acid-base imbalance 51, 53
acidosis 35
Addison's disease 49, 50, 96
adrenal gland 90, 95
adrenocorticotrophic hormone
    (ACTH) 88, 95, 96
agranulocytes 22
alanine aminotransferase (ALT)
    70–1, 75, 76
albumin 74, 76
alcohol abuse 23, 50, 83, 85
alcoholic hepatitis 71, 75
aldosterone 90
alkaline phosphatase 72–3, 75, 76
allergy 23
ammonia 74
amputation 57
androgenic sex hormone 90
anemia 15–21, 35, 36
angiotensin-converting-enzyme
    (ACE) inhibitors 49
anti-diuretic hormone (ADH) 89
aplastic anemia 19
aspartate transaminase (AST) 70–1,
    75, 76
asthma 23
atherosclerosis 82
auto-immune conditions 22, 71
auto-immune hepatitis 71

bacterial infection 22, 23
basophils 22

bicarbonate 35, 36, 63
bile duct tumors 72, 73
biliary cirrhosis 83
biliary obstruction 71–3, 75, 76
bilirubin 37, 69–70, 71–2, 75
blood
    complete blood count (CBC)
        13–29
    pH level 51
    urinary 37, 38
blood glucose 57–8, 60, 61, 62, 63
blood loss
    hypocoagulability 24
    occult 18, 20
blood urea nitrogen (BUN) 34, 35,
    59, 74
bone marrow pathology 17, 19,
    22, 23
bone pathology 73

C-peptide 61
calcitonin 89
calcium 35, 36, 49–50, 89–90,
    94–5
cancer 22, 50, 73
cardiac complications
    arrhythmia 49
    calcium levels and 50
    from diabetes mellitus 57, 63
    see also heart disease
casts, urinary 38
chemotherapy 19

Made in the USA
Lexington, KY
11 March 2015